REA

FRIENDS
OF ACPL

P9-CND-521

Disabled Rights

American Disability Policy and the Fight for Equality

Jacqueline Vaughn Switzer

Georgetown University Press
Washington, D.C.

Georgetown University Press, Washington, D.C.
©2003 by Georgetown University Press. All rights reserved.
Printed in the United States of America

10 9 8 7 6 5 4 3 2 1   2003

This volume is printed on acid-free offset book paper.

Library of Congress Cataloging-in-Publication Data

Switzer, Jacqueline Vaughn.
    Disabled rights : American disability policy and the fight for
equality / Jacqueline Vaughn Switzer.
        p. cm.
Includes bibliographical references.
    ISBN 0-87840-897-5 (hardcover : alk paper) — ISBN 0-87840-898-3
(pbk. : alk. paper)
    1. People with disabilities—Government policy—United States. 2. People
with disabilities—Civil rights—United States. 3. People with disabilities—Legal
status, laws, etc.—United States.   I. Title.
HV1553 .S95 2003
362.4'0973—dc21   2002013813

In memory of Justin Dart: 1930–2002

Gentle Warrior

Father of the Americans with Disabilities Act

Contents

Acknowledgments

Much of my interest in disability policy stems from the influence of my mother, Ruby Vaughn, who contracted polio as a child, and from my Ph.D. dissertation advisor at the University of California, Berkeley, Sandy Muir, who used braces and eventually a wheelchair. In the mid-1990s, I faced disability head-on because of my own experiences and those of my colleagues at Southern Oregon State University, several of whom unexpectedly joined the ranks of the disabled after incidents involving environmental illness. I am especially indebted to Dr. Claude Curran, who supported my efforts to bring attention to compliance with the Americans with Disabilities Act (ADA) there. At Northern Arizona University, I received two years of research support for my study of implementation of the ADA, which enabled me to do field interviews that further expanded my knowledge of disabilities and policies designed to assist people with disabilities. Dr. Edward Berkowitz of George Washington University offered initial guidance on the conceptual framework of the manuscript, as did several other reviewers. I wish also to thank Christopher Kelaher of Brookings Institution Press, who saw the potential for the book and encouraged me to continue my initial research, and Gail Grella at Georgetown University Press. She once remarked to me that "this is a story that needs to be told."

Last, I offer my gratitude to the academicians, researchers, legislators, and thousands of activists who have championed disability issues. They have framed disability policy as a subject of both political and social significance—a civil rights issue as important as any other our nation has encountered. As disability activists tend to put it, "It's the only minority group that anyone can join."

Introduction

The twenty-first century began with a series of contrasting events that illustrate both the salience of issues involving persons with disabilities and the continuing saga of discrimination that affects untold millions of Americans.

In March 2000, the Sixth District Court of Appeals overturned on a technicality the misdemeanor conviction of Kelly Dillery, who had been arrested in Sandusky, Ohio, in 1998 on a charge of being a pedestrian in a roadway. Dillery, who uses a motorized wheelchair because she has muscular dystrophy, used her wheelchair in the city's street because she said the sidewalks were raised or broken and therefore were inaccessible to her. She was charged four times in less than a year for her actions—once for child endangering because she carried her daughter on her lap (a first-degree misdemeanor for which she was later acquitted). During interviews, Dillery indicated that her daughter had learned to assist her—jumping off the wheelchair to pull her mother out of potholes in Sandusky's roadways.

The Dillery case became a cause celebre for disability rights activists. One advocacy specialist called her "our Rosa Parks" (referring to the black woman who symbolized the civil rights movement). In a rally outside Sandusky's City Hall, protestors braved near-freezing temperatures to shout, "Access is a civil right." "Her cause is all our cause," said one Ohio supporter.[1]

In May 2000, actor Clint Eastwood faced a showdown that was a far cry from the battles that characterize his film and television career. The former

I

mayor of Carmel, California, testified before the House Subcommittee on the Constitution in Washington that was considering a measure to amend the 1990 Americans with Disabilities Act (ADA). The proposal would have required plaintiffs to give defendants notice of alleged violations of the law and then ninety days to comply by taking corrective action.[2] Eastwood's testimony was a response to a lawsuit filed against him in 1997 by Diane zum Brunnen. The plaintiff alleged that when she and her husband visited the actor's Mission Ranch Inn resort, at least one bathroom and the hotel parking lot did not comply with the ADA, and there were not enough rooms that were accessible to disabled guests.

Eastwood denied that the hotel was not accessible and claimed that he was being preyed upon by money-seeking attorneys who were going after small businesses. Disability advocacy groups, such as the Paralyzed Veterans of America, supported the lawsuit and told reporters that the proposed amendment "ignores the fact that owners of properties . . . have had almost ten years to comply with the law." The amendment also was opposed by the Clinton administration, which issued a statement saying the proposal would "work to undermine voluntary compliance with the Americans with Disabilities Act and . . . unduly burden legitimate ADA enforcement activity."[3] In October 2000 a jury found Eastwood guilty of violating the ADA and required him to make his resort accessible, as well as to pay the plaintiff's attorney's fees. Ironically, the courtroom in which the case was heard was not accessible.[4]

Perhaps the most poignant comment was made by the plaintiff's attorney, Paul L. Rein. "If a black person is not allowed to enter a business because of his race, he's not required to send a letter. If a woman is not allowed to. . .she's not required to send a letter. Why should disabled persons be the only class of persons required to send letters?"[5]

In October 2000, the U.S. Supreme Court heard oral arguments in one of the most important civil rights cases of the new millennium, *University of Alabama at Birmingham Board of Trustees, et al. v. Patricia Garrett.*[6] The case involved a nurse at the University of Alabama who underwent extensive radiation and chemotherapy for a year after being diagnosed with breast cancer in 1994. She took four months of leave from work, but when she returned she was demoted and received a significantly lower salary. She filed a federal lawsuit against her employer, arguing, in part, that the university had discriminated against her while she was undergoing treatment, repeatedly threatening to transfer her or permanently replace her. She claimed that the ADA protected her against the university's actions, stating that her rights were violated when she was demoted after taking sick leave.

In federal district court, the case was consolidated with a similar case, *Ash v. Alabama Department of Youth Services.* The judge dismissed both cases on summary judgment on the grounds that the Eleventh Amendment to the U.S. Constitution grants sovereign immunity to states. The ruling had the effect of declaring that states were immune from the ADA, voiding the discrimination protections granted to disabled persons since 1990. The U.S. Supreme Court granted *certiorari* in April 2000, providing an opportunity for a critical ruling on the constitutionality of the law. The case and the Supreme Court's ruling are described in detail in the epilogue.

These events epitomize the crux of the struggle of America's largest group of citizens who are denied their basic civil rights—the more than 50 million persons in the United States with disabilities. The disability community has slowly come together in the past half-century to bring forward its demands. As with other social movements, the struggle for civil rights has meant destruction of stereotypes, attempts to capture political support, and building of coalitions among subgroups with different needs and social agendas.

George Washington University historian Edward Berkowitz begins his 1987 book, *Disabled Policy: America's Programs for the Handicapped,* with the comment, "America has no disability policy. It maintains a set of disparate programs, many of them emanating from policies designed for other groups, that work at cross-purposes."[7] Nearly twenty-five years later, Berkowitz's observation remains accurate. Despite the passage of the landmark 1990 statute, the creation of a presidential commission on the employment of the disabled, and the appointment and election of disabled activists to policymaking positions around the country, U.S. policy toward persons with disabilities (PWDs) remains fragmented. Millions of dollars are being spent on social welfare, vocational rehabilitation, and employment programs that virtually all observers agree have done little to better the lives of the disabled. The late activist Justin W. Dart, Jr., observed, "Our society still is infected by an insidious, now almost subconscious, assumption that people with disabilities are less than fully human and therefore are not entitled to the respect, the opportunities, and the services and support systems that are available to other people as a matter of right."[8]

Why is this so? This book maintains that there has been a fundamental, identifiable shift in American disability policy that can be explained only by looking at the historical context in which policymaking occurs. In the United States, there is a distinction between the medical model (or paradigm) and the civil rights paradigm—best expressed in the changeover from exclusion and humiliation to finding "cures" and a therapeutic response, to rehabilitation, to a focus on inclusion and accessibility. Disability policymaking now is based on the civil rights model, although the shift from the medical model has not been completely successful (an argument I examine throughout this book).

Other difficulties in defining, measuring, and framing disability as a public policy problem have prevented agreement on potential solutions and restricted civil rights protections. Using the passage of the Americans with Disabilities Act as a case study, the policy analysis builds on the research of social scientists like James Anderson and John Kingdon, who believe policy follows a standard progression of steps in a cycle where problems are identified, issues are adopted and solutions formulated, policies are implemented and then evaluated.[9]

DEMOGRAPHICS OF DISABILITY

Policy development has been made difficult by the lack of reliable information about the number of PWDs in the United States. Even though repeated studies have attempted to do so, there is no accurate assessment of how many individuals are disabled and what their needs are. Without that information, policymaking is based largely on guesswork rather than informed choice. How difficult is it to come up with an accurate representation of the disabled population?

The problem of demographics is complex, even though numerous public and private agencies and organizations have attempted to reach agreement on definitions and methodologies. For many years, researchers, policymakers, and the media relied on the figure of 43 million PWDs—a number alleged to have been "pulled out of the air" by a disability activist, according to one anecdotal account. Contemporary efforts have done little to improve what most observers agree are guesstimates.

One problem lies with the definition of "disabled," which means different things in different contexts, and even among agencies and statutes. The ADA, for instance, defines disability as a "physical or mental impairment that substantially limits one or more of the major life activities." Three primary terms are commonly used in determining whether a person is disabled: functional activities (seeing, hearing, speaking, lifting and carrying, using stairs, and walking); activities of daily living (ADLs), which include getting around inside the home, getting in or out of a bed or chair, bathing, dressing, eating, and toileting; and instrumental activities of daily living (IADLs) such as going outside the home, keeping track of money or bills, preparing meals, doing light housework, and using the telephone. Other definitions may be used to screen eligibility for Social Security Disability Insurance, access to social service programs, or transportation and parking placards.

The U.S. Bureau of the Census provides information on disability from three primary sources: the Survey of Income and Program Participation (SIPP), the decennial census of the population (most recently conducted in 2000), and the Current Population Survey (CPS). Each survey relies on different types of questions given to different audiences. For instance, the CPS identifies persons who are out of the labor force because of a disability and, since 1980, identifies persons who have a health problem that "prevents them from working or limits the kind or amount of work they can do." It is limited, however, to work-related data. Census forms ask only a few disability-related questions, which most often are used to compile data at the state and local levels. Because the SIPP is the most comprehensive and consistent survey of households, it is used most often in discussions of disability policy, although it is based on a limited sample and is primarily regionally based. It excludes persons living in institutions, but it does ask questions about whether respondents use wheelchairs, crutches, or canes; the presence of certain conditions related to mental functioning; the presence of a work disability; and the disability status of children, which are not part of the other two data sets.

Other government agencies, such as the U.S. Department of Commerce's Economics and Statistics Administration, note the lack of consensus on the issue of what questions should be asked to determine whether a person is disabled. The National Health Interview Survey—one of the most comprehensive sources—deals only with the prevalence of disability in the noninstitutionalized population of the United States. Perhaps one of the most respected sources on disability information, the Disability Statistics Center at the University of California, San Francisco, typically includes in its reports a series of caveats regarding limitations on the survey data it uses. The result: incomplete, often conflicting information that makes problem definition virtually impossible or, at best, imprecise.[10]

Common to contemporary discussions of disability policy is what activists call an "us vs. them mentality"—a sense that PWDs have been marginalized in society. This perception has created a new wave of militancy and, for some activists, a distrust of the promise of the ADA and subsequent policies. As one national leader put it, referring to current efforts to make facilities and programs accessible to the disabled: "We won't accept 10 percent—we want 100 percent." This book attempts to analyze that attitude and how it has led to a changing paradigm of disability in the United States.

UNDERSTANDING DISABILITY POLICY

Existing disability policies are based on a three-step shift in attitudes, values, and stakeholders. This section also elaborates on the plan of the book and its major themes. Chapter 1 begins with an overview of the policymaking process, followed by a discussion of key stakeholders (the executive branch, commissions and agencies, the legislative branch, and the judicial branch) that affect how policy is made. The book uses an institutional approach to describe what are usually termed *formal policymakers* before turning to a discussion of expressive groups and other stakeholders in later chapters.

Treatment Model

The treatment model (also called the medical model), which originated in early nineteenth century practices, was founded on policies that called for institutionalization of persons who were considered feeble, deformed, or otherwise unfit—physically or mentally. Such individuals were not only the object of public scorn and ridicule, they often were considered less than human (a theme outlined in greater detail in chapter 2). Researcher Harlan Hahn notes that this terminology "imposes a presumption of biological or physiological inferiority upon disabled persons."[11] University of Sheffield educator Len Barton goes a step further, arguing that the model "assumes an idealized notion of 'normality' against which disabled people are constantly being compared. 'Able-bodiedness' is seen as the acceptable criterion of normality."[12]

At the same time, a persistent view (and one that still attracts some support and great controversy today) is that disabilities can be "cured" and, through the modern miracles of medicine and technology, all but eliminated as a societal "problem."[13] Many disabled persons reject this perspective. David Pfeiffer, a political scientist who uses a wheelchair because of polio, remarks, "There is nothing a health care provider can do that will make us 'normal.' The problem is not the use of a wheelchair, but the concept of what is normal. People who use wheelchairs are quite normal. We are different, but normal. We have a right to be different and a right to be treated equally."[14]

Compensation and Rehabilitation Model

There is a lengthy history to the compensation and rehabilitation model (described further in chapter 3), which began just after the Revolutionary War in the United States. With the passage of state workers' compensation legislation in 1911, policies to make the disabled "financially whole" were firmly entrenched in American society. To avoid litigation, workers who were injured on the job were given various levels of financial compensation matched to specific injuries they sustained. Although levels of assistance varied from state to state, the idea of "solving" the broad range of disabled persons' needs by giving them a check was woven into the patchwork of programs that has become U.S. social welfare policy.

After the turn of the twentieth century, the emphasis broadened to provide training (now termed vocational rehabilitation) to return disabled workers to the workforce. Although this idea had been at the root of attitudes 200 years earlier, it did not become a legislative objective until 1920. Meanwhile, there were new developments in technological assistance to PWDs so that they could become part of mainstream American life. Although rehabilitation initially focused on working adults, that focus changed in 1975 with the signing of the Education for All Handicapped Children Act. Congressional studies had found that at least 1 million American children had been refused entry into public schools because of their disabilities. Chapter 3 reviews what has been called "the corrective response" and "the ameliorative response"—a series of legislative attempts to deal with disabled persons as elements of the workforce.

Civil Rights Model

Two groundbreaking statutes—the Rehabilitation Act of 1973 and the ADA of 1990—exemplify the civil rights model. Under this paradigm, the federal government mandated that PWDs be given equal access to public-

and private-sector programs, services, buildings, communication, transportation, employment, and housing.

Models are useful, however, only to the extent that they can be applied to real life. Chapter 4 provides a chronicle of disabled political and social activism over the past forty years, including the quest for inclusion that began at the University of California's Berkeley campus in the 1960s. It examines the first Center for Independent Living (established in 1972), the development of a disability advocacy movement, and attempts to create a collective identity. The chapter looks at the elements of what have been called "a fragmented social movement" and "segmented advocacy."

Unlike some other civil rights movements, advocates seeking equality for the disabled often have been working against one another. There are hundreds of disability-specific organizations, ranging from groups for persons who are deaf or hard of hearing, who have created what they term their own "deaf culture," to groups advocating for the rights of blind and visually impaired persons, to those with physical disabilities, mental and psychiatric disabilities, and cognitive and learning disabilities. Their ranks have been enlarged by the presence of groups in support of those with chronic illnesses, "invisible" disabilities, environmental illnesses, and HIV. Still others represent disabled veterans, people of short stature, children with disabilities, and disabled athletes. A representative listing of organizations appears in Appendix C. This discussion is followed by an examination of the disabled movement's strategies and leadership and the concepts of self-advocacy and cross-disability awareness. These concepts have shaped the contemporary movement's efforts at integration and, many observers believe, also have led to what writer Joseph Shapiro calls "the splintered universe" of disability.

Chapter 5 follows with a brief chronology of legislative initiatives from 1960 to 1990, focusing on amendments to disability insurance, social security laws, removal of architectural barriers, and education. That activism coalesced during the late 1980s as groups pushed forward a political agenda that culminated in the passage of the ADA, which often has been referred to as the most significant civil rights legislation in U.S. history.

Chapter 6 explores the ADA's provisions in depth, reviewing not only what the ADA was supposed to do but also what implementation studies have found it has actually done. It is a case study of policy failure and policy success, depending on the perspective of the observer.

Chapter 7 identifies and analyzes the "hot button" issues in disability policy in the twenty-first century. Eight topics are covered in detail: reproductive rights and technology, physician-assisted suicide, the role of charity telethons, the "myth of the supercrip," deaf culture and cochlear implants, the integration mandate, violence against disabled persons, and invisible disabilities. These issues have not only split the disability community, they also have led to angry protests and lack of agreement on policy goals.

Those perspectives are analyzed further in chapter 8, which attempts to provide a status report on disability. It begins with data on attitudes and the results of public opinion surveys about PWDs and how much progress is perceived to have been made. The chapter then moves on to a series of six policy issues: employment, social integration, barriers to independence, transportation, health care, and housing. In each section, the chapter examines what has been done and what remains to be done to bring about equality for disabled persons.

Finally, the epilogue looks at U.S. Supreme Court cases decided in 2001 and 2002 that have reignited debates over congressional intent and contemporary attitudes toward PWDs. The book concludes that although there are certain advantages to litigating cases that test the breadth of the ADA, activists run the risk of challenging a U.S. Supreme Court that has a much more conservative attitude toward disability rights. In those situations, coalition-building, protests, and traditional political activities are no longer useful.

A WORD ABOUT LANGUAGE

It is important to note the importance of language in understanding the complexities of disability policy. As has been the case with other social movements, words and their meanings often shape the political debate and social discourse. Just as the civil rights movements for people of color raised questions about the propriety of terms such as "chicano" and "Afro-

American," those involved in disability activism are not in agreement among themselves about terminology.

There is, of course, virtually universal agreement that pejorative terms that objectify disabled persons (such as deformed or wheelchair-bound) diminish the importance of the individual and create the perception of people only in terms of their disability. Similarly, attempts to develop euphemisms (physically challenged, height-impaired) generally are thought to be misguided attempts that still identify persons by their disability alone.[15] More militant activists have called for a return to the stereotypical terminology of prior centuries, whether the words are "cripple" or "polios." There is agreement that past attitudes need to be changed, and PWDs should attempt to develop a sense of pride, culture, and community. The use of the phrase "person with a disability," for example, recognizes that the person comes first—a human being before being someone with a disability.[16]

To some observers, the debate over language, terminology, and identity has diverted attention from more serious concerns among disabled persons. Jane West, a researcher and advocate, relates the efforts of the National Cristina Foundation to offer a $50,000 award in 1991 to the person who came up with a word or phrase that would best convey a positive empowering message about persons with disabilities. The winning phrase, "people with differing abilities," is seldom used by researchers, care providers, or those with disabilities, but no doubt it is superior to the contest entry of "severely euphemized."[17]

Although the choice may not satisfy all readers, this book attempts to use "mainstream" terminology as reflected in the literature of disability studies and scholarly research.[18] Generally, the term "handicapped" has been avoided in favor of "disabled," although the former term is still found frequently in legislative references. The book attempts to avoid obvious stereotypes wherever possible to create a level of writing that is readable and nonjudgmental. As with other social movements, however, the world of PWDs is dynamic and sometimes unstable, as reflected in the language and politics of our times. Any phraseology that is perceived as objectionable or biased is entirely unintentional on the part of the author.

CHAPTER I

Disabled Policymaking/Disabled Policy

Harlan Hahn, founder and director of the Program in Disability and Society at the University of Southern California, is a political scientist who believes that among the issues that form the current agenda of political debate, "perhaps few offer as much promise for achieving significant political change as the development of public policy affecting disabled Americans."[1] This chapter outlines how disability policy has emerged as a legitimate issue on the policy agenda, beginning with a profound paradigm shift that began in the late 1970s and early 1980s. It provides an overview of the policy process, using a model developed by John Kingdon, and the role of various stakeholders who have shaped contemporary policies leading up to the passage of the 1990 Americans with Disabilities Act (ADA).

The basic theme of this chapter is that there has been an identifiable and distinct shift in public policy—a sea change in the way programs for disabled persons are designed and implemented. Ruth O'Brien, who has studied the paradigm shift as it relates to the workplace, traces the change to the research conducted during and after World War II. O'Brien cites advances in rehabilitation medicine and the work of Howard Rusk and Henry Kessler as an important stage in this process: "Rehabilitation was promoted to ensure the health of the individual *and* that of society. According to [Rusk and Kessler], an unrehabilitated person could weaken and erode society's health."[2]

The change also is typified by a 1983 policy statement from the National Council on the Handicapped. The federal agency no longer approached a person with a disability from the perspective that such a person was someone who has been damaged or flawed, who is dependent on charity or government assistance (the treatment model and the compensation model). The council called on the government to shift to policies that achieve "maximum life potential, self-reliance, independence, productivity, and equitable mainstream social participation in the most productive and least restrictive environment."[3] This change calls for government to play a role in altering the political environment, primarily by extending civil rights.

THE PARADIGM SHIFT

Why has disability policy finally made its way to the policy agenda? Hahn notes that an important shift in the prevailing definitions of disability has led to an opening of the "policy window" described by Kingdon and others (a process described more extensively in chapter 5). Initially, disability was defined as a medical issue that focused on impairments of mobility, vision, or hearing—defects or organic conditions. As a result, persons with disabilities were placed in separate diagnostic categories, and the solution to the "problem" of disability was to improve an individual's functional capability. For the person with polio, the answer was braces or a wheelchair. For someone who was blind, service dogs or the teaching of Braille was appropriate. "As a result, the issue of disability not only was depoliticized, but the preoccupation with etiological diagnosis also fragmented the disability community by stressing the functional traits that divided them rather than the external obstacles that they faced as a common problem."[4] Hahn believes that this attitude prevented groups from rallying around issues or forming coalitions with one another—actions that would have facilitated the emergence of a broad social and political movement of citizens with various types of disabilities. At the same time, disability policy was viewed from an economic perspective related to whether a person with a disability was able to work. Other life activities were omitted from consideration.

In the 1970s, there was a profound shift in the paradigm that previously had been based on health and economics. Instead, policymakers began to look at disabled persons from the perspective of architectural, institutional, and attitudinal barriers to full participation and integration. At that point, disability began to be regarded in terms of civil rights, bias, and discrimination. Hahn believes that this shift resulted in the realization that the external world is shaped by public policy and that policies are a reflection of pervasive cultural values and attitudes.

> Structures are built, messages are transmitted, and institutions are created, primarily because laws, ordinances, and regulations permitted them to be constructed in that manner. As a result, governments bear an inescapable responsibility for those facets of the environment that have a discriminatory effect on persons with disabilities.[5]

Despite the fact that discrimination against persons with disabilities often has been compared to the discrimination faced by other minorities, however, George Washington University historian Edward Berkowitz explains why it is important to differentiate among them:

> For one thing, people are not necessarily born handicapped, unlike those who are born black or female. Nor do the handicapped give birth to future generations of handicapped or promote a handicapped culture. The lack of this common culture isolated the handicapped from each other, and the isolation was exacerbated by the fact that the handicapped differed greatly among themselves.[6]

Researchers William Johnson and Marjorie Baldwin believe there are distinct differences between people with disabilities and those who are black. "Unlike black Americans, the majority of persons with disabilities were not subject to discrimination in access to education or in employment during their childhood years," they note. "Another important difference between the black and disabled minorities is the extreme heterogeneity of prejudice towards persons with different disabilities."[7]

Berkowitz notes that one aspect of the public policy problem was how to apply the insights that had been gained from the minority model to programs for disabled persons. Doing so involved a subtle but important change in how the policy problem was framed. Some programs and services would be designed for those whose disability was called "enfeeblement" or "loss of powers one once had" that often was a product of the aging process.[8] Individuals in this category were likely to need protection against a loss of income, such as disability insurance or income maintenance programs. Other policies would be needed for those termed "handicapped" who needed "independence incentives" and protections against discrimination.

Adding to the paradigm shift were important issues raised by economists, who argued that disability policy should not be shaped by civil rights but should be developed on a cost/benefit basis—a debate that continues to complicate policymaking even today. At the time, making buildings or buses accessible was framed in terms of how many individuals would benefit, and at what dollar increment.[9] At a September 2000 conference in Washington, D.C., designed to measure the benefits of providing accessible transportation, disability activist Patrisha Wright asked rhetorically, "Would we ask what the cost/benefits are of putting black people on a bus?"

This chapter begins with an overview of the policymaking process, which subsequently is used to chronicle the development of disability policy. It identifies key stakeholders involved in making disability policy, inside and outside the formal structure of government. Elemental to the paradigm shift have been two changes: the development of social and political activism of persons with disabilities described in chapter 4.

OVERVIEW OF THE POLICYMAKING PROCESS

The policymaking process can be considered in many ways, and different perspectives have affected the development of American disability policy.

This section seeks to define that process more closely by explaining what is usually referred to as the policy cycle model of public policymaking, described and used extensively by James Anderson and John Kingdon.[10] Anderson and Kingdon bring slightly different but compatible perspectives to understanding public policy; these perspectives are especially applicable to disability policy. The application of this model is discussed in depth in chapters 5 and 6.

The key to the policy cycle model is that there is a predictable and logical sequence of activities that can be used to explain how a policy develops. Although the process is dynamic overall, in a constant state of change and movement, it also can be viewed in distinct stages.[11] Commonly, the major steps are described as follows:

1. Agenda setting
2. Policy formulation
3. Policy legitimation
4. Policy implementation
5. Policy and program evaluation
6. Policy change

Agenda Setting

In 1984, Kingdon proposed that the political system is actually three separate but interdependent "streams" of activities that flow continuously. The *problem stream* is composed of information, research, reports, and evaluations that circulate in the political environment, providing primary data on various public problems. The stream may be affected by variables such as electoral change (a presidential election), a crisis (a major protest or demonstration that is widely covered by the media), a technological development (voice-activated computer software), or other events that prompt the public to pay greater attention to the issue. When the public's interest is cohesive and strong enough regarding an issue, the problem may be made part of the *policy agenda*—which Kingdon describes as the list of subjects or problems for government officials and those who interact with government, which begin to hold their interest and to which they pay serious attention.

A second aspect, the *policy stream*, consists of proposals that begin to develop as legislators, interest groups, academicians, and others discuss potential solutions to solving the problems that are emerging. Some proposals are immediately dismissed as being too costly or impractical; others develop a political following of sorts. For instance, a plan to require the National Park Service to make all of its facilities physically accessible to persons with disabilities might be termed impractical because it would destroy the historical fabric of older buildings. On the other hand, a proposed appropriation to create an interpretive center that would showcase artifacts from a site might gain support from those involved in the decision making.

The third element, the *politics stream*, is another way of describing the political environment: public opinion, the activities of expressive groups, changing paradigms. Interest groups try to mobilize public opinion as a way of bringing about change—for example, disability rights groups used protests as a strategy when they chained themselves to buses as a way of emphasizing the fact that transportation was not accessible to them.

Kingdon's model is based on the idea that although the three streams usually flow independent of one another, from time to time they converge. That convergence usually is the result of the opening of a *policy window* (of opportunity, described more fully in chapter 5) and the presence of a *policy entrepreneur* who takes the lead on the issue. The policy entrepreneur may be someone inside or outside the formal structure of government, but it inevitably is an individual who is able to mobilize those interested in the problem to action. Anthony Downs uses a similar model to explain how the agenda-setting process also goes through a cycle.[12]

Policy Formulation

This stage is when solutions are identified, proposed, and analyzed. It generally is described as an incremental, often messy process that modifies existing policies rather than blazing new policy ground. It may involve trial-and-error decision making;[13] consideration of a very limited set of alternatives that are familiar and easily understood;[14] technical and often contradictory scientific studies;[15] and domination of public discourse by one group or another, limiting debate and idea development.[16] Policy formulation does not necessarily involve decision-making equals, and in most cases some groups are better organized and more influential than others. They may dominate the debate because they hold more political clout, financial resources, or other forms of power in the political environment.

Policy Legitimation

At this stage of the policy process, proposals are brought before the legal bodies that can approve them and then set the wheels of action into motion. Legislatures, county governments, city councils, or regional boards—usually made up of duly elected representatives—legitimize the policy because they represent constituents who have given them that power. The public usually is involved in some way during this stage as members of expressive interest groups. Citizens may testify at hearings, send letters to public officials promoting their cause, be part of a task force or planning group, and lobby their representatives. Again, not all groups have identical resources to use these strategies, so their input is not always heard or acted on.

Policy Implementation

The bureaucratic arena becomes a major part of the implementation process when government agencies, bureaus, and commissions begin the task of putting legislation into effect. Sometimes their role is very clear, especially when their legislative directives are limited or clearly defined. Often, however, the laws and statutes are intentionally vague, leaving room for interpretation and discretion. Implementation also is affected by the amount of resources provided by the legislative body. Even the most well-crafted statute may fail to be implemented if there are no funds to give agencies rulemaking or enforcement powers. This factor, too, may be intentional—and may be a result of inadequate legitimization. At this stage, agency officials decide how to prioritize their actions and what the legislative body intended the law to mean; they also are influenced by interest groups that continue to press their agendas. Implementation can be affected by the level of expertise of staff members charged with drawing up regulations, their personal desire to see the programs succeed or fail, and partisan considerations.[17]

Policy and Program Evaluation

Ideally, every government policy goes through a process in which judgments are made about how well the policy is working and whether it is meeting its objectives. This process may involve formal evaluation by Congress or another government body such as the General Accounting Office or outside investigations conducted by citizen watchdog groups. Generally, this evaluation process looks at the outcome of the policy— what has been produced, how cost-effective it has been, how many clients have been served, and plaudits and criticism from the media, the public, and those affected by the policy.[18]

Policy Change

If policy evaluation works successfully, it may result in policy change— revisions to make the policy more successful or a decision to terminate it altogether. Policy change also may be initiated by forces within the political environment. For example, a change in control of the White House or Congress, differences of opinion about whether a policy has outlived its original purpose and is no longer needed, or an attitude change toward deregulation or decentralization also may lead to policy change. Although it is somewhat rare for a government program to be eliminated entirely, it does happen.[19] Lastly, the policy may have caused unintended consequences—results that were impossible to predict even with the best attempts at planning. When this happens, policies with negative consequences may lead to policy change or termination.[20]

KEY STAKEHOLDERS

One of the best ways to deconstruct American disability policy is to examine the roles and power of key stakeholders in the political debate. Sometimes this approach is referred to as an institutional analysis because it focuses on the formal structure and legal aspects of government bodies, including the relationship among relevant institutions and actors.[21] Although this is only one methodology among many in the discipline of policy analysis, it does help to explain the role of various actors who make decisions.

Executive Branch

American disability policy—in particular, the 1973 Rehabilitation Act and the 1990 Americans with Disabilities Act—is effective only to the extent that the executive branch of government makes it so. This section provides a brief overview of agencies and commissions and their responsibilities related to persons with disabilities, their effectiveness, and their overall impact on the policymaking process. As Box 1.1 shows, dozens of federal agencies, commissions, and offices within the executive branch are responsible for implementation and enforcement of disability rights laws. The two foremost government agencies are the U.S. Department of Justice (DOJ) and the U.S. Equal Employment Opportunity Commission (EEOC). Historically DOJ has been the agency that helps citizens resolve the majority of discrimination complaints; the EEOC has focused its efforts on discrimination in employment in the public and private sectors.

DOJ has delegated its authority for enforcement to its Civil Rights Division (CRD), established in 1957 as the lead agency charged with investigating violations and discrimination in the early years of the civil rights movement for people of color. The CRD is headed by the Assistant Attorney General for Civil Rights and has authority for monitoring and revising regulations, investigating and resolving complaints of discrimination, and enforcing compliance with statutes and executive orders related to disabilities. Since the passage of the ADA, the CRD has undergone a series of internal reorganizations, transferring some of its responsibilities to four other sections within DOJ: Disability Rights, Special Litigation, Voting, and Housing and Civil Enforcement.[22] The Disability Rights Section, created in 1995, devotes virtually all of its staff time and resources to the ADA because it is the only federal agency authorized to litigate against state and local government employers.[23]

The EEOC became a key stakeholder in prohibiting discrimination in employment in 1964 as part of the Civil Rights Act. Under Title VII, the commission's mission is "to promote equal opportunity in employment by enforcing the federal civil rights employment laws through administrative and judicial actions, and education and technical assistance."[24] The EEOC deals with discrimination in the public and private sectors, although originally it could not enforce decisions of the courts without assistance from DOJ. When Congress amended the Civil Rights Act in 1972, the EEOC's authority was expanded to include the power to file lawsuits against private employers when negotiation efforts failed, and under President Jimmy Carter's 1978 Reorganization Plan the commission received additional responsibility for age discrimination and enforcement of the Equal Pay Act. Disability was not included as a form of employment discrimination until the passage of the ADA.

In 1992, when the employment provisions of the ADA went into effect, the EEOC gained considerably more power to process complaints. There is universal agreement, however, that the commission has been unable to adequately review and evaluate ADA-related complaints, as well as perform its other duties. A major reorganization in May 1997 created eleven offices within the EEOC, along with fifty field offices. Those most involved in disability policy are the Office of General Counsel, the Office of Legal Counsel, and the Office of Field Programs. The General Counsel is

BOX 1.1

Government Agencies with Responsibility for Disability-Related Programs

Federal Communications Commission
    Disabilities Issues Task Force
General Services Administration
    Center for Information Technology Accommodation
    National Program for Accessibility
    Office of Enterprise Development
Government Printing Office
Job Accommodation Network (JAN)
Library of Congress
    National Library Service for the Blind and Physically Handicapped
National Council on Disability
National Institute for Literacy
Social Security Administration
    Office of Employment Support Programs
Telecommunications Access Advisory Committee
U.S. Architectural and Transportation Barriers Compliance Board (Access
    Board)
U.S. Department of Agriculture
U.S. Department of Education
    National Institute on Disability and Rehabilitation Research
    Office for Civil Rights
    Office of Special Education Programs
    Office of Special Education and Rehabilitative Services
    Rehabilitation Services Administration
U.S. Department of Health and Human Services
    Administration on Developmental Disabilities
    Administration for Native Americans
    Centers for Disease Control, Office on Disability and Health
    Center for Mental Health Services Knowledge Exchange
    Disabilities and Managed Care
    Health Care Financing Administration

National Institute on Deafness and Other Communications Disorders
Office for Civil Rights
Office of the Surgeon General
President's Committee on Mental Retardation
Women with DisAbilities
U.S. Department of Housing and Urban Development
U.S. Department of the Interior
U.S. Department of Justice
Civil Rights Division
U.S. Department of Labor
Census Bureau
Office of Disability Employment Policy
Presidential Task Force on Employment of Adults with Disabilities
Access America for People with Disabilities
U.S. Department of Transportation
U.S. Department of Veterans Affairs
USA Jobs

responsible for all enforcement litigation; the Office of Legal Counsel provides legal advice to the chair of the EEOC and the agency itself. It includes three divisions, including the ADA Policy Division, which develops and interprets EEOC policy guidance as well as providing technical assistance. The Office of Field Programs is a service organization that also provides technical assistance and education and coordinates alternative dispute resolution.

Several other cabinet departments also have responsibility for investigating and resolving disability-related complaints: the U.S. Departments of Agriculture (USDA), Education, Health and Human Services (HHS), Housing and Urban Development (HUD), Interior, Labor (DOL), and Transportation (DOT). These seven departments represent the executive branch agencies with the largest civil rights compliance staffs and the most experience in complaint investigations and disability issues, although the level of expertise varies considerably. HUD, for example, did not open its

Office of Disability Policy until 1996—around the same time the agency itself was being sued by activist groups for failing to comply with the 1973 Rehabilitation Act.[25] There also is some overlap among these agencies, leading to a complex system of referrals of cases and investigation.

In 1977 the White House Conference on Handicapped Individuals— one of the major forums for discussions of disability policy—recommended establishment of a federal agency to coordinate programs for disabled persons.[26] The recommendation was adopted a year later with the creation of the National Council on the Handicapped as an advisory board within the U.S. Department of Education, bringing that agency into the review and evaluation process. In 1984 the National Council on the Handicapped was established as an independent federal agency (see below).

DOL became one of the major stakeholders in the executive branch in 2000 when President Clinton accepted a recommendation to create an Office of Disability Employment Policy (ODEP) within the department. In effect, the office took over the functions of the President's Committee on Employment of People with Disabilities (described below), giving disability policy cabinet-level visibility for the first time. Previously, DOL had a variety of programs whose goals were to eliminate policy barriers that impede employment of people with disabilities. Part of the office's responsibilities are to help implement the Workforce Incentives Act and the Workforce Investment Act, which make it possible for persons with disabilities to accept jobs without losing their health care benefits, and to establish a series of one-stop career centers throughout the United States.[27]

Commissions and Other Programs

In the past fifty years, almost every president has attempted to show his concern for disabled persons by creating some kind of commission or task force specializing in disability-related issues. Although the names change slightly from one administration to the next, most are showpiece panels that routinely issue reports and recommendations that call for greater inclusion of disabled persons in society, especially in the employment sector.

Aside from the cabinet departments, the executive branch also has established several other programs that share responsibility for shaping disability policy. The President's Committee on Employment of People with Disabilities was established in 1947 by President Harry Truman's executive order to encourage employers to hire disabled World War II veterans. At the time, it was called the President's Committee on National Employ the Physically Handicapped Week, and its primary activity was to promote that annual campaign. One of the group's major accomplishments was to publish reports showing that disabled employees were efficient and had low absenteeism rates, making them desirable as workers. The committee also was the source of the now universally recognized symbol for accessibility—a blue profile of a person in a wheelchair. In 1962 it became the President's Committee on Employment of the Handicapped as a way of broadening its clientele to include those with developmental and psychiatric disabilities. Over the succeeding twenty years it became an advocacy agency, sponsoring meetings with congressional leaders in support of the 1973 Rehabilitation Act and the right of persons with disabilities to have access to airlines, subways, and buses.

In 1989 President George Bush appointed longtime disability rights advocate Justin Dart, Jr., to head the committee. Dart promptly changed the name of the organization to the President's Committee on Employment of People with Disabilities and refocused its attention on monitoring legislation, research, and creating a network of state-level committees. It provided technical assistance on the ADA after its passage, disseminated public service announcements, developed two employment demonstration programs, and sponsored the Business Leadership Network to interest more employers in hiring disabled workers.

In 1998 President Bill Clinton continued the tradition of presidential involvement but put his own symbolic stamp on the issue with the creation of a National Task Force on Employment of People with Disabilities, chaired by the Secretary of Labor.[28] In this incarnation, the membership included the heads of several cabinet departments and other federal agency officials. The goal of the task force (renamed the President's Task Force on the Employment of Adults with Disabilities), like its predecessors, was to develop federal policies to reduce employment barriers faced by persons with disabilities. In 1999 President Clinton and Vice President Al Gore announced a multifaceted initiative to implement the recommendations made by the group, including funding for the 1999 Work Incentives Improvement Act, provision of a tax credit for work-related expenses for people with disabilities, and expansion of access to information and communications technologies.[29]

Tony Coelho, a former member of Congress from California who was active in legislative efforts to enact the ADA, served as Dart's successor on the President's Committee on Employment of People with Disabilities. The committee's responsibilities were subsumed by DOL in October 2000.

One type of disability has received special consideration within the executive branch. In 1961 President John F. Kennedy, responding to his family's experiences with mental retardation, appointed a special President's Panel on Mental Retardation. The group was composed of physicians, educators, members of the parents' movement, and psychologists who surveyed existing programs and treatment methods. In 1962 the panel released 112 recommendations, including more comprehensive and improved clinical services, resulting in passage of the Maternal and Child Health and Mental Retardation Planning Amendments a year later.[30] This legislation and a companion statute, the Mental Retardation Facilities and Community Mental Health Centers Construction Act,[31] were considered landmark steps to provide funding for research into the causes and prevention of mental retardation.[32] The panel disbanded in 1962 but was reconstituted in 1966 by President Lyndon Johnson in the form of the President's Committee on Mental Retardation. It was expanded in 1974 by President Richard Nixon and continues to issue conference proceedings and reports emphasizing deinstitutionalization, as well as assistance for children and families.

An independent federal agency, the National Council on Disability (NCD) (as noted above, originally the National Council on the

Handicapped), is made up of presidential appointees and was conceived in 1978 in amendments to the Rehabilitation Act as an advisory board in the U.S. Department of Education. Although the NCD has the mandate of tracking enforcement of the ADA, it has no power or staff to accomplish that goal. Instead, it provides policy and program reviews, makes recommendations to the president and Congress, sponsors conferences and forums, and publishes an annual report on disability policy.[33] One of its most valuable contributions was a 1986 report that called for civil rights protection for persons with disabilities, which became part of the groundwork for the drafting of the ADA.[34]

Finally, the National Institute on Disability and Rehabilitation Research (NIDRR) began operation in 1978 as the National Institute of Handicapped Research, and now provides technical assistance for implementation of the ADA. Primarily an information clearinghouse, the NIDRR oversees the activities of regional centers, develops reference materials and speakers/trainers, and helps bring together other disability policymakers. Its programs are funded by federal grants.

Legislative Branch

Although expressive interest groups brought their concerns to members of Congress in the early stages of the battle for disability rights, congressional interest faded when the ADA was signed on July 26, 1990. The legislative leaders in the fight for passage of the law are described in greater detail in chapter 5. One congressionally chartered group, however, was afforded an opportunity to shape disability policy: the Task Force on the Rights and Empowerment of Americans with Disabilities, created in May 1988 by representative Major Owens of New York. Owens served as chair of the House Subcommittee on Select Education when it was one of the four subcommittees deliberating the proposed ADA. The task force, which received no public funding, was chaired by Justin Dart, Jr., and included prominent disability rights activists. It became the means by which individuals and groups across the nation gave members of Congress their input on the

proposed statute. All fifty states held hearings—sixty-three in all—and
more than 5,000 documents were included in the task force's final report,
released in October 1990.[35]

Judicial Branch

Prior to passage of the ADA, cases of discrimination involving persons with
disabilities seldom found their way into the judicial arena—and deliber-
ately so, for several reasons. For complaints arising under the ADA and
Section 504 of the Rehabilitation Act, for instance, there are several phases
of complaint processing that require grievances to be submitted in writing
on standard forms. Complaints may be closed if they are incomplete or
if the complainant does not respond with requests for additional information. Because the DRS receives many more complaints than its staff can
handle, many are not "opened" as cases to be investigated.[36]

The associate director of the Illinois Department of Human Services has
criticized the DRS for its lack of staff and delays in the processing of complaints: "The ADA is limited mainly by the inability of those agencies
responsible for enforcement to act in an expedient manner. . . . The major
policy issue is the slow manner in which ADA complaints are dealt with."[37]
Even cases that do warrant investigation must then go through a time-consuming process of reviews, complaint summaries, documentation, and—
very rarely—referral to the U.S. Attorney, whose office also may decide not
to proceed with the action. This sifting process leads to only a handful of
cases being investigated, let alone adjudicated.

To ease the backlog of complaints and the extended processing period,
program analysts within DRS make a determination about whether the
matter is appropriate for alternative dispute resolution or mediation. With
a technical assistance grant, the Key Bridge Foundation trains professional
mediators on the requirements of the ADA; the DRS does not directly
mediate cases. About 2–3 percent of cases have been handled in this fashion, keeping them out of the court system. In fact, a section of the ADA
requires that DOJ attempt to negotiate a resolution of complaints before

starting litigation.[38] In one sense, litigation becomes a final resort, and in the majority of cases actually filed, a complaint is resolved at the time a suit is filed or soon afterward. The mechanism used, a negotiated consent decree, is a judgment between the parties in which the defendant agrees to stop the illegal activity without admitting guilt or wrongdoing.

This area of implementation has come under sharp criticism by disability rights activists, who believe that precedents that will be binding in subsequent cases will be established only through the courts.[39] As noted in chapter 6, however, there has been an increasing trend toward taking "major" cases to the courts as a way of building visibility for the ADA and perhaps giving notice to those who discriminate against disabled persons that they face the threat of litigation now more than ever.

CHAPTER 2

History of Segregation and Stereotypes

Many scholars have attempted to find ways of deciphering the history of disability policy, using arbitrary benchmarks or relying on legislative milestones to mark the various phases of attitudinal and policy development. Others have concentrated on the language of disability as a way of explaining societal treatment of persons with disabilities. This chapter seeks to provide an overview of the values and attitudes that have become part of the political environment in which American disability policy has evolved over the past 100 years.

One of the earliest models of social disability, developed in 1948 by Jane and Lucien Hanks, uses a five-part typology to explain the participation of disabled people in selected non-Western societies. *Pariahs* are persons who are denied all claims to relief by society and are deemed a threat to the group itself. *Economic liability* is the phrase used to describe the perception that disabled people are unwelcome because they are thought to drain resources or deflect attention from other needs. *Tolerant utilization* refers to situations in which disabled people are "allowed" to participate in societal activities when it is deemed appropriate by those who are not disabled. In contrast, *limited participation* implies that there are situations in which a disabled person can "blend" into society by meeting the norms and standards of the dominant majority. Last, *laissez-faire* situations are those in which society provides support for working and nonworking disabled per-

sons. It does not imply, however, that there is any attempt at accommodation or social equity for disabled persons.[1]

The terms *normal* and *abnormal* also have been used to distinguish persons with disabilities, lending a normative spin to their context in societal terms. Researcher Simi Linton notes that these terms move discourse
"to a high level of abstraction, thereby avoiding concrete discussion of specific characteristics and increasing ambiguity in communication. In inter-
actions, there is an assumed agreement between speaker and audience of
what is normal that sets up an aura of empathy and 'us-ness.'"[2]

Robert Funk describes the evolution of disability history and policy in
four time frames that he believes represent the increasing humanization of
disabled people. In the United States, he cites the period from 1700 to 1920
as a time when extended families provided care for disabled persons; when
societal indifference produced abuse, state-funded institutions were created to house indigent disabled citizens. Phase 2, from 1920 to 1960, was
characterized by segregation, the growth of rehabilitative medicine, and
the establishment of special organizations that attempted to educate the
public on the needs of disabled persons. The third phase, from 1960 to
1975, is marked by the development of the disability rights movement and
federal statutory reform. After 1976, disability organizations expanded,
while a changing political climate and a conservative executive branch produced what is regarded as a generally restrictive interpretation of disability rights law.[3]

Although these models are useful, if simplistic, the history of the development of disability policy is much richer and more complex than most
Americans realize. In one sense it is aligned with the development of other
civil rights movements, but there also are important differences that this
book attempts to explore. Much of the complexity is found in changes in
attitudes toward disabled persons—a process that has been glacially slow
at best.

Perhaps the word that best describes the historical treatment of persons
with disabilities is *separation*. Although in some cultures the family takes
responsibility for the care of disabled persons, for the most part this has

been the exception rather than the rule in the United States. More commonly, disabled persons have been isolated, institutionalized, and ignored. In the first half of the twentieth century, persons with disabilities were treated as "freaks" and exploited. Many families sold their disabled children for exhibitions; sideshows were common throughout Europe and the United States, with impresarios such as P. T. Barnum bringing carnivals and circus dime museums to cities large and small.[4]

About the same time, some efforts were made to provide care for people who were considered "unfit or enfeebled." In Europe, religious groups housed disabled children and orphans; in nineteenth- and twentieth-century America, asylums were set up for people who were unable to care for themselves. For most of recorded history, however, the world has made it clear that persons who are physically or intellectually different do not belong with the rest of society. The tendency also has been to use pejorative labels and to stereotype persons with disabilities, ignoring the individual and concentrating instead on the disability.

Even before the United States gained independence, disabled people were separated from the general population and their condition equated with poverty. The Duke of York (who in 1665 governed territory that is now portions of New York, Pennsylvania, New Jersey, and Delaware) declared that disabled persons should be subject to the charity of the region's citizens, later combining disabled and indigent people as a single group. Another statute required that indigent and impotent persons wear a large Roman "P" on the shoulder of the right sleeve of their garments, in an open and visible manner.[5] Pennsylvania enacted statutes in 1729 that allowed public officials to deport persons with physical impairments.

In the early nineteenth century, charitable groups in the United States established institutions designed primarily to care for children, beginning with the American School for the Deaf in Hartford, Connecticut. Thomas Gallaudet, who had studied methods of teaching deaf children in France, founded the school (then the Connecticut Asylum for the Education of Deaf and Dumb Persons) in 1817.[6] Fifteen years later,

Boston's Perkins School for the Blind (originally called the New England Asylum for the Blind), modeled after institutions in Europe, admitted its first two students. In 1848 the Perkins Institution, as it was then known, opened the first residential facility for people with mental retardation. These organizations took responsibility for the care of disabled persons at a time when neither state nor federal policymakers felt obligated to do so.

Several social reformers attempted to convince policymakers to fund some form of publicly funded "relief," especially for children. In Massachusetts, the state legislature named Samuel Gridley Howe head of a commission to study "the problem of the feebleminded," which resulted in a legislative appropriation in 1849 that created the Massachusetts School for Idiotic Children and Youth in Boston. Although Howe initially intended that youth would attend the school to gain life skills and then return to their families, many parents felt that their children were better off staying at the facility and refused to take them back.[7] As a result, segregation became the norm and institutionalization the means for society to keep unwanted individuals out of the mainstream.

Dorothea Lynde Dix also attempted to change the government's attitude toward disabled persons, but the emphasis remained on institutionalization. Dix spent two years in England, where she witnessed firsthand the inhumane treatment of persons with mental disabilities. In the United States, most mentally disabled persons ended up in poorhouses, jails, and prisons (thoroughly chronicled in a survey Dix conducted in Massachusetts). Although Dix was able to convince Congress that federal funding should be provided to support state hospitals for mentally and physically disabled persons, she could not gain President Franklin Pierce's support for the measure, and he vetoed it in 1854.[8] Sociologist Richard Scotch notes that these early institutions were "founded with great hopes for improving society. In the decades that followed, however, efforts at rehabilitation and social reform proved to be overly optimistic. Institutions took on an essentially custodial nature, overladen with the rhetoric of reform," rather than educational purposes.[9]

"The Problem of Feeblemindedness"

A second phase of attitudinal development—the use of labeling and stereo-types—began just before the start of the twentieth century. The stigma of mental illness, which often was confused or associated with chronic illness such as epilepsy, led to many abusive practices and procedures. Clifford Beers, who later became a pioneer in the early disability rights movement, attempted suicide in 1900 because he believed he had inherited his brother's epilepsy. Initially taken to a Connecticut asylum, Beers spent three years in three different institutions and in 1908 chronicled his experiences in his book *A Mind that Found Itself.*[10] Beers documented the brutality and sexual assaults that were routine in mental facilities and surreptitiously kept records on the lack of heat and clothing and the over-medication of those confined to them. After the book was published, Beers founded the Connecticut Committee for Mental Hygiene, which in 1909 became part of the National Committee for Mental Hygiene.[11]

James Trent, Jr., who has studied the history of mental retardation in the United States, notes that there was a profound shift in policy in the 1840s as feeblemindedness, or idiocy, began to be regarded as a social and state problem rather than a family and local problem. The shift can be traced largely to the work of French educators Edouard Seguin and Dr. Felix Voisin, whose two institutions in Paris were considered models for the care of persons who had been neglected as uneducable. Similar schools (many of them private) were later opened in western Massachusetts and near Albany, New York, by Hervey Wilbur, a young physician who also was impressed by Seguin's work. Philadelphia's citizens opened a private school in 1853; this example was followed by Ohio in 1857, Connecticut in 1858, Kentucky in 1860, and Illinois in 1865.[12]

A second change that occurred prior to the turn of the twentieth century was the shift from the educational model (training) to a medical model that considered retardation from a pathological, typological, and degenerative perspective. Dr. Linus Brockett, for example, in an influential article in the *American Journal of Education* expressed his view that there was a pathological basis for feeblemindedness, although he fell short of actually calling the condition a disease. "We should define idiocy," he said, "as the result of an infirmity of the body which prevents, to a greater or less extent, the development of the physical, moral and intellectual powers."[13]

Another change in the framing of disability as a "problem" and, later, as a policy issue came when many American reformers, in a departure from the French, began to regard idiocy as a hereditary condition. In the early 1900s, psychologist Henry H. Goddard, using his research on what would later be known as intelligence tests, attempted to create a linkage between disabilities, immorality, and crime. Goddard alleged that disabilities were a result of genetic weaknesses that were passed from one generation to another; he used the term "moron" to describe those who were permanently mentally deficient. At least two-thirds of all feeblemindedness, Goddard believed, was the result of hereditary factors or the "cancerous growth of bad protoplasm."[14] This position also changed how society regarded persons who were considered mentally deficient. No longer merely a social burden, they became a social menace.

Goddard soon proposed that feebleminded individuals be tested to determine their intelligence level, then either placed in segregated institutions or prohibited from marrying and, if necessary, sterilized. His views gained public support in 1912 after the publication of his book *The Kallikak Family: A Study in the Heredity of Feeble-Mindedness*.[15] The book traced the family tree of a young girl who had been a student in one of the institutions where Goddard and his assistant, Elizabeth Kite, had worked. Kite used a questionable methodology to show that the girl's idiocy and degeneration could be traced back to forebears living at the time of the American Revolution, who eventually produced 143 feebleminded offspring, along with epileptics, prostitutes, alcoholics, and criminals. Goddard used the family's story to show that there was a direct causal link between vice and mental retardation.

The Kallikaks were not the only family to be chronicled as examples of hereditary degeneracy, however. They were joined by the Jukes,[16] the Nams,[17] and other contemporary studies of families called "defectives," usually living in poor, rural areas.[18] The stereotypes continue to this day with jokes and comments about families living in close proximity to one another and cases of intermarriage.

Goddard's theories were important in the development of disability policy for two major reasons. First, they spawned support among the American public for institutionalization on an unprecedented scale. In 1890 there were twenty public and four private institutions in the United States for the care of individuals termed morons—a population estimated at 5,254. By 1903 there were twenty-eight public and fourteen private facilities housing 14,347 individuals, building a trend toward lifelong institutionalization.[19] Second, feeblemindedness became associated with the massive levels of immigration that had begun in the latter part of the nineteenth century. By 1917 Congress was considering a measure that would ban the immigration of "persons of constitutional psychopathic inferiority," reflecting what James Trent refers to as "a growing fear of defective strangers."[20]

Twentieth-century public policy toward physically and mentally disabled people was shaped by the growing eugenics movement. Eugenics—a term coined by British mathematician Sir Francis Galton in 1883—is defined as "improving the quality of the stock."[21] Supporters of the movement believed that white, heterosexual, able-bodied Protestants of northern European descent were the pinnacle of human evolution, and all others (including nonwhites, homosexuals, and especially people with disabilities) were not only inferior but also threatening to the survival of the species as a whole. Prior to World War II, there were close linkages between the American and Nazi eugenic movements.[22] One German film, distributed to more than 3,000 U.S. high schools, described people with disabilities as "weeds" who needed to be cut away so that the healthy might survive.[23]

Eugenics also was an outgrowth of the industrial revolution of the mid-nineteenth century, when the term "feebleminded" was applied to anyone who was unable to reach a minimal (third-grade) educational level. Although the term often was applied to persons who today would be considered learning disabled, virtually anyone who was unable to attend a regular public school also was stigmatized, including those with mobility, speech, or vision impairments. That tendency, described as "spread" by Beatrice Wright and others, remains prevalent today. Wright explains the concept as follows: "People are likely to take a single characteristic of a person, such as a physical disability, and infer another trait such as an inability to learn or to make intelligent decisions. . . . Having a disability is too often equated with being feebleminded."[24]

The eugenics movement gained considerable support from about 1890 until the 1940s, led by advocates who opposed the social welfare programs of the 1930s and anti-immigration sentiment. Around the turn of the twentieth century, xenophobia toward nonwhites and people with disabilities reached its zenith, according to historian Kenneth M. Stampp. These groups were lumped together in the category of "unassimilable aliens," and the "solution" was state-imposed segregation.[25] The similarity between the Jim Crow laws of the South and the prejudice against disabled people has been noted by several authors, most of whom cite policymakers' belief that such segregation at the time was considered benign and beneficial.[26]

The most common remedy suggested to deal with "the problem of feeblemindedness" (aside from extermination) was voluntary or, if necessary, forced sterilization. One writer cautioned, "No feebleminded person should be allowed to marry or become a parent. . . . Certain families should become extinct."[27] In 1927 the U.S. Supreme Court reinforced what had become standard practice in most states, ruling 8–1 in *Buck v. Bell* that forced sterilization of people with disabilities who were wards of the state was constitutional. The case involved Carrie Buck, a seventeen-year-old girl who was a resident of the Virginia Colony for Epileptics and Feeblemindedness. Prior to being taken to the facility, Buck had been raped by a member of her foster family, and officials ordered her sterilized on the grounds of "moral imbecility." Without even performing any examination of Buck or her mother, a determination was made that both women belonged to "the shiftless, ignorant, and worthless class of antimonial whites of the South."[28] Writing for the Court, Chief Justice Oliver Wendell Holmes wrote that "it is better for all the world, if instead of waiting to execute degenerate offspring from crime, or to let them starve for their imbecility, society can prevent those who are manifestly unfit from continuing their kind."[29] Between 1921 and 1964 an estimated 63,000 persons were sterilized involuntarily in the United States for some "genetically related reason,"[30] and although the state legislation that led to the *Buck* case was repealed in 1968, forced sterilization continued for several more years in some states.

Assistance and Treatment

Well-meaning and often well-educated social workers and reformers attempted to ameliorate the brutality of institutions and the separation mentality by developing tools that would help persons with disabilities live independently. In 1860 Simon Pollack of the Missouri School for the Blind brought a new communications aid to the United States. A system of raised letters and symbols that could be "read" had been developed in France by Louis Braille and later modified by American educators. As often has been the case with the introduction of new technology, however, policymakers argued among themselves over various versions of Braille until 1910, when "American Braille" was adopted as a standard by the American Printing House for the Blind. The language's use remains controversial even today as computerized scanners and portable cassette recorders have reduced the number of persons who actually use Braille to read.[31]

Perhaps the most recognizable aid for disabled persons is the wheelchair. The U.S. Patent Office registered the first design for one in 1869, and a folding model was patented forty years later. Bulky, expensive, and cumbersome, the early models provided some mobility for persons with physical disabilities, but it was not until the 1970s and the advent of wheelchair sports that designs were radically altered. In addition to the lighter weight, racing bike-styled "Quickie," power wheelchairs provided freedom for persons with spinal cord injuries, multiple sclerosis, or other severe disabilities. Unfortunately, while technology moved forward, public policy did not. The availability of such devices remains limited by public funding for health care, insurance carriers attempting to keep the cost of durable medical goods down, and distribution. Moreover, getting a wheelchair is one thing; making a home accessible or finding transportation that can be adapted to accommodate wheelchair users is something else.

Persons who are deaf or hard of hearing have faced a struggle similar to that faced by those who are blind or have limited vision. In the mid-nineteenth century, Bernard Engelsman founded the New York Institution for the Improved Instruction of Deaf Mutes. Using a system he had learned in Vienna, Engelsman began teaching students to read lips and attempt speech. His "oral school" used techniques (oralism) that were the antithesis of the manual or sign language method advocated by Gallaudet and others. Advocates of the two competing approaches battled for scarce resources, and many schools forbade their students from using what had become known as American Sign Language, or ASL. It took decades for ASL to gain acceptance, and its use remains controversial among some members of the deaf community.[32]

"Treatment" procedures became as controversial as policies to provide assistive devices, especially after media reports flourished that focused on the abuse of persons with disabilities who were being institutionalized. Public attention was captured to some extent in 1946 by the riveting account of life in public mental institutions in Mary Jane Ward's *The Snake Pit,*[33] which was made into a film in 1948, and *Christmas in Purgatory*, a photographic documentation of brutalizing conditions that was published in 1966.[34] By the late 1960s, terms such as "mainstreaming," "normalization," and "residential care" had begun to replace institutionalization in state facilities, which gradually were being shut down.

Debates over treatment continued through the rest of the century, however. Psychotropic medications—known derisively as "chemical straitjackets"—were developed at the turn of the twentieth century to make people with mental illness more docile and compliant. Yet the use of mind-numbing drugs, along with aversive therapy, remains the treatment of choice in many institutions today. Aversive therapy, for example, often is used to control the actions of people with developmental disabilities, and corporal punishment is common. Disability rights activist Nancy Weiss has documented treatment in U.S. facilities that she equates to that afforded political prisoners.[35]

The contemporary horror of inadequate institutional care is exemplified by what came to be known as "The Willowbrook Wars." The term refers to a series of events that took place at New York's Willowbrook State School, which opened in 1951. Advocates for disabled people provided hundreds of accounts of insufficient medical care, neglect, malnutrition, improper sanitation, forced seclusion, and abuse that resulted from cuts in state funding and poor staffing. An ABC television report in 1972 that showed naked children lying in their own waste and filthy conditions at the facility led to massive protests by parents and eventually a class action lawsuit on behalf of the residents that reduced the size of the facility's population from 5,400 to 250; most of the former patients were placed within community care.[36]

The Willowbrook experience was part of a major change in disability policy—deinstitutionalization—that attempted to bring an end to the warehousing of disabled persons.[37] In 1962 a President's Panel on Mental Retardation commissioned by President John F. Kennedy recommended the development of a wider range of alternatives for people with developmental and psychiatric disabilities.[38] A series of landmark court cases led justices to rule that conditions in institutions were so cruel as to be considered unconstitutional and that people with developmental disabilities had a right to live in the community.[39]

THE STEREOTYPES CONTINUE

Just as the landmark case of *Brown v. Education* in 1954 failed to produce immediate desegregation of the nation's public schools, passage of nondiscriminatory legislation has failed to put an end to the stereotypes that still characterize persons with disabilities. According to several researchers, the problem lies with the media, which have pigeonholed disabled people into common stereotypes. "There is the sad, unlucky disabled person, in need of pity and charity. Or there is the plucky, courageous disabled person, celebrated for overcoming a disability and performing seemingly superhuman feats, whether holding a job or scaling a mountain. One is the image of Tiny Tim, the other that of the 'super crip.'"[40] In the words of writer Joseph Shapiro, who has covered the disability rights movement in depth, these stereotypes have slowed progress toward full inclusion in American life. "To be seen as patient or in need of charity is to be thought incapable of the same life as others. To be lauded for super-achievement is to suggest that a disabled person can turn our pity into respect only at the point of having accomplished some extraordinary feat."[41]

These images represent a pattern of what researchers Robert Bogdan and Douglas Biklen call "handicapist stereotypes"[42]—seven images used commonly by the media in its depiction of persons with disabilities:

1. *The disabled person as pitiable and pathetic.* This form of continuing negative stereotyping is found in charity telethons, which perpetuate the image of people with disabilities as objects of pity. Their stories often are told in terms of people who are victims of a tragic fate, rather than a social minority.

2. *The disabled person as Supercrip.* These heartwarming stories, says journalism professor Jack Nelson, depict great courage—or what is often referred to as "disability chic"—wherein someone likable either succeeds in triumphing or succumbs heroically. The problem, one observer notes, is that a lot of ordinary disabled people are made to feel like failures if they haven't done something extraordinary. Disability advocates are exceptionally harsh and critical of such individuals and their "inspirational" coverage.[43] (This topic is explored further in chapter 7.)

3. *The disabled person as sinister, evil, and criminal.* In this stereotype that plays on deeply held fears and prejudices, the disabled villain—espe-

cially one with a psychiatric illness—is almost always someone who is dangerous, unpredictable, and evil. This perception may lead to unwarranted apprehension and ostracism of people with disabilities, robbing them of their sense of self by regarding them only as exemplars of a stigmatic trait.

4. *The disabled person as better off dead.* Nelson refers to the "better dead than disabled syndrome" as one way in which the media implies that with medical costs soaring and resources limited, a disabled person would seek suicide because life often is unbearable. Society (or the family) is thereby relieved of caring for the disabled individual, who is not whole or useful.

5. *The disabled person as maladjusted—his or her own worst enemy.* "If only disabled persons were not so bitter and would accept themselves, they would have better lives" is the translation of this common stereotype. Usually it involves a nondisabled person who helps someone with a disability see the "bright side" of his or her impairment—the mythology that persons with disabilities need guidance because they are unable to make sound judgments.

6. *The disabled person as a burden.* Family responsibility and duty form the core of this stereotype, which is built on the assumption that persons with disabilities need someone else to take care of them. Like the stereotype of disabled persons as better off dead, it engenders the belief that the burden, whether financial or emotional, is so compelling that it ruins families and their lives. In contemporary parlance, it has focused on the hot-button issue of physician-assisted suicide described in chapter 7.

7. *The disabled person as unable to live a successful life.* The media has distorted society's views of what it means to be disabled, according to Nelson, by limiting the presence of disabled persons in the portrayal of day-to-day life. Although more disabled people are beginning to appear in cameo-like scenes, they are seldom seen in workplace situations or as happy, healthy family members. This legacy of negative images is both damaging and inaccurate.[44]

What is important about these enduring stereotypes, however, is the fact that they have helped frame the policy debate over the civil rights of disabled persons. Richard Scotch notes that the legal precedents for protecting PWDs against discrimination came primarily from the Civil Rights Acts of 1964 and 1968. Both statutes were clear in their goal of protecting individuals facing discrimination because of their race. In the case of disabled persons, however, policy initiatives were made for different reasons: a perceived societal obligation to provide for dependent disabled persons and the assumption that there would be benefits to society from making disabled individuals economically and socially self-sufficient.[45] That difference in goals and objectives is the subject of chapter 3.

CHAPTER 3

Compensation and Rehabilitation

A merican disability policy has at its foundation a series of social welfare programs that can be traced back to the nation's earliest history.
What is most important in analyzing the early attempts at policymaking
is that those programs have never been integrated into a holistic approach
that considers not only the differences among disabled persons but the lack
of cohesiveness among the programs that do exist. The lack of planning
and coordination have almost always been referred to in pejorative terms:
"isolated," "piecemeal," "incoherent."

The second of the three models used to describe the development of
American disability policy is based on the concepts of compensation and
rehabilitation. In this model there is an assumption of governmental
responsibility for providing financial consideration to disabled persons and
an attempt to make the body "whole" through rehabilitation. The former
approach has been called the *ameliorative response* to disability because it
provides financial assistance to disabled persons without dealing with disability itself.[1] By redistributing income, the government simply transfers
money without making any attempt to change the disabled person's ability to work or become a part of the larger society. In one sense, this
approach "sentences" the disabled person to a lifetime of welfare payments
(and more important, health benefits) with little likelihood of change. It
is at the heart of most contemporary workers' compensation programs,

44

as well as social security disability insurance, which are the focus of the first half of this chapter.

In contrast, Robert Haveman and others consider vocational education and rehabilitation part of the *corrective response* to disability policy. Instead of providing financial compensation, the corrective response focuses on improving the productivity of disabled workers, providing assistive technology or devices to help them overcome impairments, or otherwise improving their economic environment.[2] Researcher Edward Berkowitz likens this approach to an investment. Instead of transferring funds to an individual whose condition is not expected to improve, an investment approach to disability may even save money because the disabled person may gain employment or improve his or her job status and income.[3] The goals also are different: dependence versus independence.

This chapter begins with an overview of the ameliorative response by providing a brief history of compensation to disabled people, followed by the development of programs to aid those injured in industrial settings and the modern workers' compensation program. A second approach—social security and, more specifically, disability insurance—is another way of making transfer payments to compensate persons who are disabled. The second half of the chapter looks at corrective responses: vocational education, rehabilitation, and education of disabled children. An analysis of the growth of rehabilitation as a part of the business end of disability policy follows, and the chapter ends with a summary of the provisions of the 1999 Ticket to Work program.

HISTORICAL BASIS OF COMPENSATION

Compensation for work-related injuries has its roots in the Revolutionary War, when prevailing attitudes of "usefulness" were tied to a man's ability to do productive work. Initially, the young nation established a public policy of taking responsibility for soldiers who were wounded in the war. When the nation's need for soldiers was acute, even those who had been injured were expected—and in some cases compelled—to continue to help defend the country. When the need for soldiers was reduced, those who were injured were regarded as "useless," and the government's responsibility was limited solely to their maintenance. Over time, this perspective developed into a tradition that the value of physically abnormal people was limited to the degree that their ability to work was limited.[4]

The public policy response began with the passage of the Pension Act of 1776, which provided compensation for individuals who had a service-connected disability. A year later, a resolution created a Corps of Invalids, using disabled soldiers as instructors in a school for propagating military knowledge and discipline. Wounded soldiers also served as recruiters and guards for the Army. A second legislative measure—An Act for the Relief of Sick and Disabled Seamen—was enacted by Congress in 1798, creating the Maritime Hospital Service, which would later become the U.S. Public Health Service. Each of these initiatives was bound to the country's desire for freedom from foreign domination (especially on the high seas) and reinforcement of the dominant political economic structure.

In the early nineteenth century, the government continued its policy of compensating its warriors by providing funds for veterans of the War of 1812 and the 1835 Mexican War. In addition to money, the government gave injured soldiers grants of land as compensation. Coverage was expanded to their wives in 1836 through the Widows' Pensions Act. The benefits were further expanded through the General Law of 1862, which would later cover veterans of the Spanish-American War and the Boxer Rebellion.

Pensions were first paid to disabled veterans of the Civil War in 1862. Two years later, the Corps of Invalids was renamed the Veteran Reserve Corps; it comprised soldiers who were disabled in combat while in service to the Union Army. Their duties included guarding Confederate prisoners of war, forming honor guards, and defending railroads throughout the occupied South. Even then, however, disabled soldiers were separated and assigned uniforms that were a lighter shade of blue than those of other units.[5] After the war, the veterans became a powerful political force, organizing as the Grand Army of the Republic.

The first private pension plan for disabled workers was adopted by American Express in 1875. It provided benefits for employees who were older than age sixty and had worked at least twenty years for the company but who could no longer work. At the state level, the first state to provide pensions for blind persons was Ohio, which enacted a statute in 1898.

After World War I, the nation faced another challenge of dealing with the wounded as they returned from battle. Many public health agencies and hospitals were unsure about how best to deal with so many veterans. Their answer came in the form of vocational rehabilitation (discussed later in this chapter).

INDUSTRIAL-RELATED DISABILITIES

The industrialization of the United States in the twentieth century brought with it a need to provide health care for the millions of workers who were employed by railroads, shipping, and the timber and mining industries, as well as the general population. In many workplaces, employees were exposed to serious health and safety risks, but few had any form of health care or occupational safety protection. Businesses that were essential in fueling the Industrial Revolution went unregulated for years because of the political and economic power of the controlling industrial leaders.

What little assistance there was in these industries was provided by the private companies themselves. Medicine was controlled by corporations; the railroads alone hired 6,000 surgeons to treat sick and disabled workers. "Employers had economic incentives to keep skilled laborers healthy and on the job, working at high levels of productivity, while also restricting liability and insurance costs and capturing the goodwill of employees and the public. Such a system also served their own interests."[6]

Industrial injuries presented a different problem than individuals who became disabled as a result of service in the military. The idea of workers' compensation was borrowed from Germany, Finland, and Austria, where legislative plans for compensating workers injured in industry had been developed toward the end of the nineteenth century. In the United States, reformers and union leaders pushed for state laws that held employers directly liable for injuries to employees, although workers had to sue the employers in court to be compensated. Maryland was the first state to enact a workers' compensation law (in 1902), but two years later it was declared unconstitutional. It was not until 1911 that Wisconsin and New Jersey began to shift responsibility by enacting no-fault workers' compensation, which Berkowitz has referred to as "the nation's first modern disability program."[7] By 1929 workers' compensation laws were in effect in all but four states.

The marketplace responded by offering employers insurance to cover potential losses, and as demand grew coverage became more costly to purchase. As part of the Progressive reform movement, social activists began to seek stronger workplace protection and safety laws for employees. The resulting melange of state-level administrative programs and the use of the courts for dispute resolution led to a more adversarial process, however, rather than the informal one reformers had envisioned. The courts became clogged with cases that took years to resolve, and more often than not state industrial accident commissions were administered by incompetent or corrupt officials. Attorneys found willing litigants among immigrants, hustling clients in hospital waiting rooms and at the scenes of industrial accidents.[8]

SOCIAL SECURITY

The compensation model also has been the basis for the United States' preeminent social welfare program—social security. The term "social security" was first used in 1933 when the American Association for Old-Age Security became the American Association for Social Security. Major events in the development of social insurance programs are outlined in Box 3.1.

In an address to Congress on January 4, 1935, President Franklin D. Roosevelt called for legislation to provide assistance for the unemployed, the aged, destitute children, and the physically handicapped. The three programs that originally were covered by the federal government when the president signed omnibus legislation on August 14, 1935, were welfare payments, unemployment compensation, and old-age retirement. The intent at that time was to bring together and coordinate widely disparate policies that operated virtually independent of one another. States, for example, were in charge of unemployment compensation; the federal government funded, but let states administer, welfare; old-age insurance was under federal auspices. Only commercial and industrial workers were covered under the latter program, which began paying out pensions in 1940—two years earlier than had been planned. The only disability specifically covered under the 1935 law was blindness, and there was no serious congressional debate about covering other forms of disability.[9]

The Social Security Board—renamed the Social Security Administration (SSA) in 1946—began the task of determining eligibility for disabled persons in the mid-1930s. Deciding whether someone was disabled was considered "conjecture" by Arthur Altmeyer, who headed the agency from 1936 to 1953. Program administrators complained that it was impossible to determine who was permanently disabled and who was facing temporary disability. The result was a definition that had been utilized by the War Risk Insurance Act, which defined disability as an "impairment of mind or body which continuously renders it impossible for the disabled person to follow any substantial gainful occupation, and which is founded on conditions which render it reasonably certain that the total disability will continue throughout the life of the disabled person."[10]

As Berkowitz notes, the SSA's definition of disability became more flexible between 1936 and 1948, as the agency attempted to consider not only the individual's impairment but also the personal, economic, and social circumstances of the time. "Variables considered relevant included sex, race, urban or rural residence, occupation and experience. The inclusion of these variables implied that disability insurance would act as a safety net into which marginal labor force participants could fall."[11] The discretion given to officials who were forced to make a determination about eligibility, however, also made the program considerably more complex. It also equated old age and retirement with disability, which then emphasized

BOX 3.1

Key Events in Development of Social Insurance Programs for Persons with Disabilities

1789   Federal government accepts responsibility of providing pensions to disabled veterans of the Revolutionary War

1798   Congress establishes Marine Hospital Service to provide medical care for sick and disabled seamen

1875   American Express establishes first private pension plan for disabled employees

1897   Minnesota becomes first state to provide medical and surgical aid for crippled children

1898   Ohio passes first law to provide pensions for blind persons

1902   Maryland enacts first workmen's compensation law; law is declared unconstitutional in 1904

1908   Workers' compensation program established for civilian employees of the federal government

1911   Wisconsin enacts first workers' compensation law to be ruled constitutional

1917   First grant-in-aid programs for vocational rehabilitation enacted through federal legislation

1920   Smith-Fess Act passes Congress to provide vocational training and counseling programs for civilians injured on the job

1933   First use of term "social security"

1935   President Roosevelt calls on Congress to provide assistance for unemployed persons, destitute children, aged persons, and physically handicapped persons; Social Security Act becomes law

1950   Social Security Act Amendments establish program of aid to needy persons who are permanently and totally disabled

1956   Social Security Act amended to provide benefits to permanently and totally disabled workers ages fifty to sixty-four

1972   Social Security Amendments establish Supplemental Security Income (went into effect January 1, 1974)

1980   Social Security Amendments provide greater work incentives for persons with disabilities

1984	Congress enacts Disability Benefits Reform Act
1999	President Clinton signs "Ticket to Work" bills to increase employment among those who wish to work
2002	States begin implementation of "Ticket to Work" program

income maintenance (the compensation model) rather than returning the individual to work (the rehabilitation model).

Administrative tinkering with the social security system continued until World War II, when the subject became problematic as the policy priorities of the nation shifted. Disability insurance was a drain on a troubled economy that needed additional funds to support the war effort. After the war, the political situation was even less conducive toward repackaging of a national disability insurance program. In 1948, a congressionally enacted advisory council took up the issues of permanent disability insurance, coverage for workers younger than age fifty-five, dependents' benefits, and the cost of the overall program. The cost estimates (which ranged from $15 million in 1950 to a half-billion dollars by 1970) were overshadowed by concerns that a less restrictive eligibility system would expand the entire program.[12]

Concurrently, opposition to disability insurance began to build. Members of the American Medical Association worried that passage of such a comprehensive program would lead the country down the road to national health insurance. Furthermore, the group argued, it would serve as a disincentive to rehabilitation, granting workers a check instead of encouraging them to try to return to work. The organization supported complete elimination of disability insurance in favor of vocational rehabilitation. Similar objections were raised by the National Association of Life Underwriters and the National Association of Manufacturers.

In 1950, Congress passed legislation in the form of Aid to the Permanently and Totally Disabled, making clear its intent to distinguish between types and levels of disability. The states were to be given control over the funds and allowed to decide who would be eligible for benefits. To many observers, this approach made perfect sense because the states already made determinations on eligibility for public assistance, workers' compensation, and vocational rehabilitation. The 1950 legislation seemed to be a natural extension of existing programs. In reality, however, it led to a patchwork system of inequality and discrimination because the eligibility standards varied from state to state.

During the Eisenhower administration, political maneuvering colored the disability insurance debate, although the focus remained on rehabilitation rather than compensation. The Republican administration opposed legislation that would have expanded coverage while its own officials in the SSA were lobbying members of Congress for its support. Under the leadership of Senate majority leader Lyndon B. Johnson, Congress expanded benefit coverage through Social Security Disability Insurance (SSDI). On August 1, 1956, President Eisenhower signed the disability insurance program into law, with applications accepted beginning in October 1956 and payments beginning in July 1957. Benefits were available under the same definition of disability that had been the backbone of social security programs: An applicant needed to show evidence of a medically demonstrable impairment that precluded gainful activity for at least a year. However, only persons ages fifty to sixty-four were covered by the law, and the states would continue to determine eligibility for benefits and administer the law. (The age threshold was repealed in 1960.) Under SSDI, disabled persons were allotted benefits on the basis of how long they had worked and how much they had contributed to Social Security through their paychecks.

A second major change in disability policy occurred in 1972 when Congress created Supplemental Security Income (SSI), although the program was not operational until January 1, 1974. Under SSI, extended benefits were available to persons who had become disabled prior to age twenty-two and had never been able to work. However, the program required beneficiaries to meet a "needs test" that determined whether their income met a predetermined threshold for eligibility. Most important, the program allowed persons with disabilities to be covered by Medicaid after two years of SSDI benefits. Although some provisions were made to encourage rehabilitation and the purchase of adaptive equipment that would allow a person to return to work, many individuals did not want to take advantage of those aspects of the program because it would mean they would lose Medicaid coverage. Yet the financial compensation alone left most disabled persons living below federal poverty levels.

The Disability Insurance Crisis

In the early 1970s, social security programs went through a period of tumult as the size of the aging population increased and benefits rose because rates were tied to inflation. The result, as many policymakers could easily see, was a system that was paying out more in benefits than it was taking in from workers' paychecks. In addition, the most costly of the programs was disability insurance. Entitlement programs came under sharp attack as critics argued that for many workers it was almost as advantageous to rely on disability insurance payments as it was to work for a living. Rather than being a last resort for indigent people, disability insurance was perceived as a federal giveaway. Making the problem even more complicated was the fact that many recipients of disability insurance benefits also were able to receive other forms of social welfare, with little coordination of benefits among state and local programs.

From a purely economic standpoint, persons with disabilities did gain substantially in terms of the benefits they received from the mid-1960s to the late 1970s. From 1968 to 1978, the number of recipients of public disability transfer programs as a percentage of the employed workforce grew from 9.3 percent to nearly 15 percent—a 7 percent annual growth rate in this period. Over the same period, expenditures for disability income support programs grew from 5.8 percent of federal government spending to 8 percent—a 6.3 percent average annual rate of growth. The sharp increase was regarded by some observers as a red flag for policymakers, who sought to restrain the growth of recipients and expenditures. The result, under the administration of President Jimmy Carter, was that the SSA notified officials that application of the rules for determining a person's disability needed to be tightened up. By 1980, the growth rate among recipients and expenditures had begun to decrease.[13]

With the advent of the Reagan administration, cutbacks in social welfare programs overall were reflected in federal support for disabled persons. SSDI, for instance, was reduced from 3.1 percent of overall social welfare expenditures to about 2.5 percent between 1980 and 1987. Much of the decrease can be credited to the Social Security Disability Amendments of 1980, which called for a review of eligibility every three years. The goal was to make regular determinations about whether beneficiaries were capable of returning to work, but implementation of the act was impersonal and often without any medical review. A lack of qualified staff to review recipients' conditions allowed many cases to go unchecked. Yet even after a General Accounting Office (GAO) audit cautioned authorities that many recipients who were taken off benefits would appeal the decisions and win, the Reagan administration moved forward to "purify" the disability rolls.[14] Within a two-year period, 838,000 recipients had their cases reexamined, and 360,000 were dropped from the rolls—many designated as "recovered" from being disabled without ever having been evaluated in person.

At the heart of the process were extremely optimistic estimates of how much money would be saved by the reviews. The Office of Management and Budget (OMB) referred to "bad management" of the program and said that as many as 584,000 ineligible beneficiaries were receiving benefits. The potential savings, OMB said, could amount to $50 million in fiscal year 1981 and $1.1 billion by fiscal year 1986. As the reviews began, the SSA increased its estimate of dollars saved to a half-billion dollars in fiscal year 1983.[15]

It was not until 1984 that the Senate and the House unanimously passed legislation that enabled about two-thirds of the recipients who had been dropped from the program to re-enroll under the Social Security Disability Reform Act of 1984.[16] The legislation was a response to thousands of individuals who had requested an appeal of their termination of benefits. Advocacy organizations such as the Alliance of Social Security Disability

Recipients, the Disability Rights Center, and others contacted members of Congress with horror stories about individuals who waited more than a year for review of their appeal.[17] The 1984 statute was in complete contrast to the 1980 version, protecting individuals from being dropped from disability insurance rather than finding ways to get them off. "In the end, disability insurance became a more secure entitlement for those who managed to get it; the coordination of programs and the reform of the disability system remained as elusive as ever."[18]

VOCATIONAL EDUCATION

Just before World War I, the nation's leaders increased their support for vocational education for young people—a policy that would set the stage for the military's response to the thousands of wounded soldiers returning from the war.[19] The Commission on National Aid to Vocational Education was established in 1914 to deal with escalating school dropout rates and a generation of young adults who were unprepared to join the workforce. Low productivity made the United States economically vulnerable and noncompetitive, so vocational training was used to upgrade workers' skills. After the war, Congress enacted legislation that would provide for the 250,000 service members who would eventually attempt to return to civil employment. One author has noted the utilitarian attitude of the government toward disabled soldiers. "A vocational rehabilitation program that would turn soldiers into economically useful civilians apparently was seen both as an expression of gratitude and as a method to benefit the national welfare."[20]

This corrective response is essentially an effort to reduce dependence on government assistance by improving worker productivity or removing barriers (physical, attitudinal, and programmatic) that hinder self-improvement and access. Berkowitz argues that this model holds "the promise of saving the government money and of returning money to society in the form of an impaired person's productivity."[21] Policymakers have not always agreed, however, on the goals of rehabilitation per se. One observer believes that "the goal of rehabilitation should be to help each person achieve in life whatever life adjustment that person is capable of attaining"[22]—an overly broad definition that provides little direction to public officials.

In 1920 an attempt to develop a more narrow definition was implemented through the Vocational Rehabilitation Act to include "persons disabled in industry or in any legitimate occupation," leading to a debate about the proper role of the federal government.[23] Many advocates argued that federal assistance to individuals who were injured on the job was "a moral obligation consistent with the nation's traditional values," whereas others contended that the legislation was "a cheaper and more economical plan than . . . keeping them in the poorhouse or in sanitariums."[24] By 1921 thirty-five states had adopted programs, and by 1932 forty-four states had begun to provide assistance to disabled civilians, each with its own criteria for the eligibility of rehabilitants. The emphasis remained on segregation, however, with disabled vocational trainees separated from other trainees. The goal was vocational assimilation into the workforce, not social assimilation.[25]

Although the workers' compensation program and vocational rehabilitation were envisioned as working hand-in-hand, they approached disability from two different perspectives. The workers' compensation bureaucracy had always been aligned with employers, unions, and agencies whose primary function was to monitor workplace safety and working conditions. Administration of these programs usually came under the aegis of state-level industrial commissions, with the federal Department of Labor (DOL) as overseer.

In contrast, the heart of vocational rehabilitation was its focus on education; consequently, state-level school officials (who also had responsibility for administration of local schools) were given additional mandates with little additional funding. Most vocational rehabilitation programs initially were administered by the Federal Board for Rehabilitation Education, an independent agency after World War I. Control was then shifted to the Department of the Interior; then to the Department of Health, Education, and Welfare (HEW); and then to the Department of

Education when it became a cabinet-level agency within the executive branch. In the early 1950s, labor unions supported a final move that placed vocational education under DOL, finally aligning workers' compensation—the ameliorative response—with the corrective response of vocational education. The Office of Vocational Rehabilitation, which had been made a separate office of the Federal Security Agency, was moved again to HEW in 1953.

At issue was whether two such differently focused programs could really provide for the varying needs of disabled people. The objectives of the two programs were different, and they were continually competing for funding. The uneasy relationship was fueled by a lack of communication among agencies and the "creaming" of clients—attempting to help first those who needed the least amount of assistance. The greatest increase in clients was a result of welfare, crowding vocational rehabilitation services out of the picture as President Lyndon Johnson expanded his War on Poverty. Another reorganization placed the Office of Vocational Rehabilitation under the Social and Rehabilitative Services Administration within HEW when the cabinet agency underwent reorganization in 1967.

By the time the Reagan administration took over, social welfare programs such as vocational rehabilitation were no longer in favor. A downturn in the economy, coupled with expenditures for other entitlement programs, left program administrators hustling for an ever-decreasing share of federal funds. Vocational rehabilitation was considered a "fringe" program that had emerged from the 1970s only to find that it was no longer an important element of social reform. Berkowitz notes that the real value of federal funding for vocational rehabilitation decreased 31 percent between 1974 and 1982, and funding for rehabilitation of welfare beneficiaries disappeared altogether in 1982.[26]

Nevertheless, the government attempted to "sell" vocational rehabilitation as part of its assistance package, especially to disabled veterans. The Department of Veterans Affairs—which had been given cabinet-level status, in large part because of political concerns after the Vietnam War—told veterans that vocational rehabilitation is "your key to an independent future."[27] Yet the government's promises of assistance did little to help disabled people. At least three audits by the GAO found that the department was being mismanaged and that its employment placement rate for disabled veterans was very low.[28] Part of the difficulty with the program appeared to lie with the agency's inability to motivate the people it was attempting to serve—a problem that also has yet to be solved by other vocational rehabilitation programs.[29]

1973 REHABILITATION ACT

Richard Scotch, who has compiled an extensive history of the politics surrounding the 1973 Rehabilitation Act, begins by noting that attempts to extend civil rights to disabled persons by amending the 1964 Civil Rights Act were hampered by the political environment of the time. In 1972 legislation was introduced in the Ninety-Second Congress by Representative Charles Vanik and Senators Hubert Humphrey and Charles Percy that would have included physical or mental handicaps as categories of illegal discrimination. Humphrey, who had long been known as a champion of social justice, said, "That this is their constitutional right is clearly affirmed in a number of recent decisions in various judicial jurisdictions."[30] No hearings were ever heard on the bills, however—in part, Scotch believes, because of opposition from advocates who were already committed to protecting the rights of blacks.[31]

Between the creation of the Social and Rehabilitation Service under Lyndon Johnson and the presidential election of 1972, Congress took a different look at the renewal of vocational rehabilitation legislation. Based on the input of groups such as the National Rehabilitation Association and led by Senator Alan Cranston and Representative John Brademas, Congress laid down the gauntlet to President Richard Nixon with regard to social reform. One version of the Rehabilitation Act of 1972 sought to remove the program from the Social and Rehabilitation Service and place it under HEW. Severely disabled persons were to be prioritized for services under a newly created Rehabilitation Services Administration, incorporating independent living services as a way of transitioning disabled people into the community rather than the workforce. President Nixon used the pocket veto to kill the measure, but the new Congress approved an almost identical act in March 1973 after protestors from the disability rights group Disabled in Action (DIA) demonstrated at the Lincoln Memorial in Washington, D.C., and took over Nixon's reelection headquarters in New York. DIA had been founded in New York in 1970 as one of the first of the grassroots disability rights organizations and later would be the first to file suit under provisions of the Americans with Disabilities Act (ADA) to force the owners of the Empire State Building to provide ramped access to the observation tower.

In 1973 President Nixon vetoed the legislation a second time, arguing that it created too many new programs, was too expensive, and went too far in including disabled persons in the decisionmaking process. When the new Congress revised the bill a third time to meet Nixon's objections, it was eventually enacted and signed into law on September 26, 1973— becoming what one observer calls "historic in its scope and depth."[32]

Of particular attention to disabled people was the fact that the bill used an enhanced definition of rehabilitation that required the federal government to address the issue of societal discrimination. It also provided grant money for vocational rehabilitation programs operated by public or non-profit agencies; directed the National Institute of Handicapped Research to fund additional research, prioritized services for individuals with the most severe disabilities; appropriated funds for a National Center for Deaf-Blind Youths and Adults; and, under Title V, committed the federal government to providing equal opportunity to qualified workers with disabilities. Title V required executive agencies and departments to submit plans designed to increase the number of employees with disabilities, established the Architectural and Transportation Barriers Compliance Board to enforce the 1968 Architectural Barriers Act, and included most federal contractors under affirmative action plans.

The most important section of the statute was Section 504, which actually is only a single sentence at the end of the statute. It had not been a part of the original deliberations on the bill, and neither Congress nor disability rights advocates seemed to be aware of the implications of the addendum, which had been drafted by an aide to Senator Jacob Javits. It reads: "No otherwise qualified handicapped individual in the United States, as defined in section 7(6), shall, solely by reason of his handicap, be excluded from participation in, be denied the benefits of, or be subjected to discrimination under any program or activity receiving Federal financial assistance." One researcher believes that Section 504 was largely symbolic[33] because it did not apply to the private sector; the National Council on the Handicapped later noted that "confusion and inconsistency have resulted, not so much about the goal, but from the historical and continuing failure to structure and administer some Federal laws and programs in such a way as to reflect and further the national goal."[34] One activist, however, had a totally different perspective, pointing out, "It is Section 504 that contains the greatest promise. . . . Virtually every area of modern American life is inexorably intertwined with federal financial assistance and this is why the protection Section 504 offers is so important. It offers the one unifying key to mainstreaming of the disabled population into the general community on all fronts in a cohesive and orderly manner."[35]

When implementation of the legislation began, problems arose almost immediately. In 1977 HEW—which was responsible for defining Section 504—issued the first set of regulations under the statute. The rules required that all new facilities built with federal funds be made accessible within two months, with extensions for major structural renovations. The regulations also included public schools, colleges, and universities. Enforcement and compliance monitoring were delegated to the U.S. Department of Justice (DOJ). To force public entities to apply the law, grassroots organizations began to train advocates to interpret the regulations, holding Section 504 workshops across the country.

It became clear, however, that many recipients of federal funding would comply only if forced to do so. This resistance led to a wave of litigation that narrowed the scope of several vague terms in the regulations. Two of the phrases that seemed to be the most difficult to interpret were "reasonable accommodation" and "undue hardship." The former term related to the kinds of physical changes to be made in buildings or workplaces to allow full access by persons with disabilities, such as a ramp or widening of a door. What did Congress intend? In *Southeastern Community College v. Davis,* 442 U.S. 397 (1979),[36] the U.S. Supreme Court ruled that "reasonable" meant that any modifications could not impose any undue financial and administrative burdens. Almost always, the phrase was applied to changes and costs incurred by employers in accommodating their employees.

"Undue hardship"—a phrase that was used to help entities that argued that implementation costs were too expensive—had no statutory parameters. Although many advocates agreed that the intent was not to bankrupt agency budgets, there was no way of knowing how substantial a financial hardship a change had to be to be classified as "undue." The statute defined the term as "an action requiring significant difficulty or expense," which included factors such as the overall financial resources of the entity; the types of operations engaged in; and, of course, the cost. Usually this meant scrutiny on a case-by-case basis. What might be assumed to be an undue hardship for a small city, for instance, might not be considered significant for a state agency to comply with.

Both phrases later became cornerstones of the discussion over the provisions of the ADA because the proposed law would go beyond Section 504 by including private entities—a much larger group of facilities and employers than had been covered under the 1973 law.

EDUCATION FOR DISABLED CHILDREN

Although there is a historical basis for the care and education of disabled children, as explained in chapter 2, the law itself never prevented discrimination in education of disabled children. One source estimated that by the mid-1970s, at least 1 million children in the United States were being excluded from public schools because of their disabilities. Half of those children were routinely excluded from any kind of educational services that would be considered appropriate for their disability. Although a strong parents' movement had arisen during the late 1960s and early 1970s to fight for inclusion of disabled children in the public schools, the majority of disabled students were placed in "special" education programs rather than being included in the regular curriculum.[37] Parents claimed that such practices constituted segregation in the same sense that children of color had been denied equal opportunity in the classroom. Most disabled children were considered too disabled to participate in school sports, music and art programs, or other extracurricular activities.

What changed that view came, once again, from litigation. In *Mills v. Board of Education,* 348 F. Supp. 866 (D.D.C. 1972) and *PARC v. Pennsylvania,* 324 F. Supp. 1247 (E.D. Pa. 1971) the courts ruled that the state had a responsibility to provide retarded children with an "appropriate" program of education and training. In the *Mills* case the plaintiff, a twelve-year-old boy, was considered a behavior problem and had been excluded by his District of Columbia school. Using the argument that the cost of educating disabled children was not a justifiable reason for excluding them from public school, the courts relied on Fourteenth Amendment guarantees of due process in both cases to require the schools to end discrimination.

In 1975, largely as a result of the efforts of organizations such as the Association for Retarded Children, the Education for All Handicapped Children Act was passed almost unanimously by Congress as a way of responding to the earlier court decisions.[38] Signed by President Gerald Ford in 1975, the law took effect in 1978. A key phrase in the statute guaranteed all children with disabilities a "free, appropriate public education," regardless of the nature or extent of their disability. School districts were required to integrate disabled children into mainstream classrooms and to train their teaching staffs to accommodate the needs of disabled children. Procedurally, each child was to be provided with an individualized education program, drawn up by the child's teachers and parents, that eliminated the one-size-fits-all approach that had characterized disabled education prior to 1975.

School districts, which lobbied against the bill's passage because of cost, lost out to parents who met individually with members of Congress. These parents sought not only integration of their children into the school system but also funding for additional programs such as speech therapy, accessible transportation, and counseling. The administration received an estimated 27,000 letters about the revised bill. Congress responded to its constituents by making federal funds available to assist the schools, while also recognizing their limited resources. As a result, school districts were only required to provide educational opportunities that were roughly equivalent to those available to nondisabled children.

As with other civil rights laws, the education statute immediately became the subject of litigation in the federal courts. In one case, the court ruled that a school district that was unable to provide services for a child with multiple disabilities would have to seek and purchase alternative services. The concept embodied in the litigation was *inclusive education*—a much more flexible approach to educating disabled children than mainstreaming had been.[39]

The statute was expanded in 1986 to include disabled children ages three to five, and in 1990 it was renamed the Individuals with Disabilities Education Act (IDEA).[40] The law prioritized services for children with the most severe disabilities, such as autism, and included an individualized family service program similar to that provided under the 1975 law.

Two advocacy groups—the Association for the Severely Handicapped (TASH) and the Mighty Alliance for Independence Now (MAIN)—rallied in Washington, D.C., in October 1998 to protest the failure to implement IDEA. They argued that the legislation had produced "special segregation" because federal law rewards districts that provide separate facilities for children with disabilities, in violation of the law. IDEA mandates inclusion of children with disabilities to the maximum extent appropriate except when the nature or severity of the disability of the child is such that education in regular classes with the use of supplementary aids and services cannot be achieved satisfactorily.[41]

In Arizona parents resorted to lawsuits, filing a class action against the state's Department of Education. They alleged that the state had failed to deal with their complaints regarding special education services and that there was no enforcement when schools were found to be at fault. More than 1,000 parents had filed complaints in four years, yet the department did not review the complaints in a timely fashion. A federal judge ruled in the parents' favor. The court ruled that complaints must be investigated within three days of receipt and that parents must be notified of their legal rights; schools that do not follow the state's recommendations will have their funding withheld.[42]

Education of children with disabilities remains one of the most volatile issues within the disability rights movement, fueled by activist parents who are willing to fight and litigate when necessary. Although some school officials may consider legislation such as IDEA interference in their right to local control of education, parents are convinced that unless the schools are prodded and monitored, the laws will not be effectively enforced.

DISABILITY AS A BUSINESS/REHABILITATION AS AN INDUSTRY

Researchers such as Gary Albrecht have focused on one additional approach to compensation and rehabilitation that often is an ignored aspect of American disability policy: the elaborated disability as business model. Albrecht notes that in this model, business managers and shareholders regard persons with disabilities as the focal point of a business defined by medical and rehabilitation professionals; government officials; and, to some extent, consumers. Each of these stakeholders has become part of an industry—a process that happens when a group of companies or organizations emerges in the marketplace, offering the same services or products. Albrecht argues that reconceptualization of disability as a business and emergent industry is important for five reasons that influence disability policy.

First, this model represents part of the paradigm shift from caring for disabled persons as a charitable activity on the fringe of the medical arena to dynamic businesses that now trade on the nation's stock exchanges. Second, the business of caring for disabled people can best be understood by realizing that rehabilitation is reimbursement-driven. Profits, cash flow management, and domain control explain as much about rehabilitation as do medical needs and technological advances. Third, the United States' role in the professionalization of health care services and the growth of pharmaceutical and hospital supply companies have tended to standardize goods and services produced in the global marketplace. Fourth, there are increasing pressures to define rehabilitation as a product and to hold providers accountable for outcomes as the financial investment in rehabilitation has grown. Fifth, intense, competitive financial pressures now affect the way rehabilitation services are delivered.[43]

Albrecht goes on to explain how important the size and growth of the disability business have become. Not only have the costs of federally provided programs skyrocketed, but private-sector businesses have become major players that can influence policy decisions affecting the entire health care debate. More and more facilities are becoming privately owned, with investors eager to cash in on the growth in the number of persons seeking some form of palliative care. The potential for market growth and profit making also has attracted foreign health care firms, and the demand for high technology rehabilitation care has brought in additional capital and investors.

"Because hospital and rehabilitation facility utilization is a function of physician referral," according to Albrecht, "these institutions strengthened their market positions by offering a broad rehabilitation product line attractive to both referring physicians and their patients."[44] Specialized programs, ranging from physical therapy clinics to home health care programs, were created specifically to meet market demand by disabled patients. The first of the for-profit, nationally oriented companies was International Rehabilitation Associates; it was followed by Crawford Rehabilitation Services and a host of other firms established in the late 1960s and early 1970s. Mergers and acquisitions, such as the mini-industry known as National Medical Enterprises, made many companies a major force in the health care field.

Parallel to the development of rehabilitation services was the growth of nursing homes and various types of community care facilities, marketed not only to disabled clients but also to elderly persons. Most of these facilities are private-sector, for-profit entities that offer some form of extended care and, more recently, hospice care, long-term care, and outpatient services. To control costs, the disability business has spun off home health care, sheltered workshops, adult day care, and respite care.[45]

The result is a symbiotic relationship among political and financial interests made up of pharmaceutical companies and medical equipment suppliers, hospitals and institutional facilities, medical consultants, insurance companies, and attorneys, all of whom share organizational linkages and affect disability policy. Sometimes their interests are altruistic, as with charitable organizations such as the Salvation Army, the American Red Cross (which set up vocational rehabilitation programs in Army hospitals during the Civil War), Goodwill Industries, and the National Easter Seal Society. Others form synergistic relationships—for example, health care organizations such as the Hospital Corporation of America, which manages and partially funds academic medical centers in Kansas and Oklahoma.

As Albrecht concludes, however, the dominant for-profit orientation of the rehabilitation industry means that the financial health of institutions and return on investment are as important as rehabilitation outcomes in treating persons with disabilities. "A growing tension exists, then, between the for-profit pressures of rehabilitation institutions and the needs of consumers with disabilities. In some instances, these forces meet; in others, they are in conflict."[46]

TICKET TO WORK AND WORK INCENTIVES IMPROVEMENT ACT OF 1999

On December 17, 1999, President Bill Clinton signed legislation that marked the next major stage in the development of American disability policy. At the prodding of disability rights groups and veterans' organizations, Congress enacted the Ticket to Work and Work Incentives Improvement Act of 1999. Several provisions in the legislation affected persons with disabilities:

- Starting in February 2002, Social Security and SSI disability beneficiaries in thirteen states receive a "ticket" that can be used to obtain vocational rehabilitation, employment, or other support services from an approved provider of their choice. Twenty more states and the District of Columbia were scheduled to be phased into this program in late 2002, with the remaining states and territories joining in 2003.
- Starting in October 2000, Medicaid and Medicare coverage was expanded to cover more people with disabilities who work, ending the need to choose between health care coverage and employment.
- Effective January 1, 2001, when a person's Social Security or SSI disability benefits have ended because of their earnings from work, beneficiaries can request reinstatement without filing a new application.
- Congress directed the SSA to establish a community-based work incentives planning and assistance program to disseminate information and give beneficiaries more choice. The agency also was required to establish a corps of work incentives specialists for persons with disabilities who want to work, with a provision that protection and advocacy systems in each state could provide information, advice, and other services to persons with disabilities.

Still untested, the Ticket to Work program marks a return to the focus on returning PWDs to the workforce. The difference between this policy and previous policies is the emphasis on choice—allowing individuals to choose what type of training or setting is best suited to their needs. The Ticket to Work statute is similar in intent to the proposed Medicaid Community Attendant Services and Support Act, which would allow similar choices in community care or assistance. President George W. Bush signed an executive order in 2001 directing federal agencies to swiftly implement the Ticket to Work Act initiated by his predecessor. Disability advocates hoped the president would look equally favorably on the Medicaid Community Attendant Services and Supports Act (MiCASSA) and implementation of the ADA as well, as will be explained in more detail in chapter 6.

CHAPTER 4

Social and Political Activism

On March 6, 1988, a silent but powerful revolution began on the campus of Washington, D.C.'s Gallaudet University. The campus, which had been founded under a federal charter in 1864 as the Columbia Institution for the Deaf and Blind, was closed down for six days in a protest led by student demands of "Deaf President Now!"—or DPN, as it came to be known. Earlier in the day, the university's Board of Trustees had announced its selection of Elisabeth Ann Rinser as the new president—a decision that not only would rock the university itself but would change the image of disability activism forever.

The protest resulted from the fact that after nearly 125 years, the trustees had once again chosen a hearing person as president of the university. The first woman selected as Gallaudet's president, Rinser was chosen over two deaf men, I. King Jordan and Harvey Corson. The board's decision was predicated on the assumption that they would choose the individual best suited for the job. Students and their supporters operated under a totally different belief system, however—one that demanded that the individual would also be deaf. To many of these advocates, Rinser's appointment was a cultural slap in the face not only because she was a hearing person but because she had no experience with deaf culture and did not know American Sign Language.

During the week's protests students demanded Rinser's resignation, as well as that of the chair of the university's Board of Trustees, and called for a majority of the board's seats to be held by deaf people. They also demanded that there be no retaliation against those involved in the protest, including students and faculty. Rinser was burned in effigy by students, as were press releases announcing her appointment. Students closed off the entrances to the campus and marched from the campus to the White House and the Capitol. A week later, the board capitulated and agreed to all of the protesters' demands, later naming Jordan as president. Rinser served only two days as president of Gallaudet before she resigned.

Two factors make this example particularly important in the history of American disability policy. First, the Gallaudet protests received worldwide coverage—an unusual occurrence for anything involving disabled people. As several authors have noted, this was more than simply a student protest—it garnered support from people of all ages and from those who were not disabled. Years later, the protest maintained symbolic visibility, making President Jordan a powerful figure in the passage of the ADA. Second, analysis of the media's coverage of events focused on the themes of self-determination and overcoming oppression rather than the kinds of stereotypical images generally associated with persons with disabilities discussed in chapter 2. One observer compared the coverage to that afforded the civil rights protests of the 1950s and 1960s, noting that the media were favorable to the protesters and communicated the idea that deaf people were a minority group.[1] Others have noted that the DPN protest was "a major contributor to the reframing process that had to occur before the ADA could become the law of the land. During DPN, media coverage showed the students as being healthy, bright, articulate, and attractive young people for whom their disability was secondary."[2]

Despite this incident, however, it is important to note that the political and social activism of persons with disabilities differs slightly from other social movements and civil rights struggles. First, no single individual or group can be identified as the leader of the disability rights movement and the policies the movement is attempting to shape. There is no Martin Luther King, Jr., or National Organization of Women to serve as the unified voice of disabled persons (a phenomenon that is explained in depth later in this chapter). Second, the rise of a disabled rights movement has gone largely unnoticed by other minorities, most Americans, the media, and many policymakers. Indeed, the laundry list of civil rights struggles often fails to include disabled people at all. This phenomenon is unusual given that researchers such as David Meyer and Sidney Tarrow believe that we are now part of a "social movement society."[3]

This is not to say, however, that the political and social activism of the disabled rights movement that led to the passage of the ADA is entirely unlike that of other groups. This chapter begins with a brief overview of the types of expressive interest groups that have been active in the formation of American disability policy, followed by a discussion of the primary strategies used by disability rights activists. It concludes with the observation that in many ways disability policy has been shaped by strategies that for the most part are traditional forms of social and political activism.

Disability Rights as a Social Movement

Much of the scholarly research on social movements comes, not surprisingly, from the discipline of sociology. Within sociology there are several competing theories about how social movements can be conceptualized, how beliefs coalesce, how resources are mobilized, and how social scientists can quantify movement successes and failures.[4] One of the more common definitions is that a social movement is a collectivity acting with some continuity to promote or resist a change in the society or group of which it is part.[5] There also is some agreement that a social movement has a sustained political agenda, that its members have a group identity, and that some form of leadership hierarchy is needed to guide the movement.

There is some disagreement about whether disabled persons fit into the social movement typology because they do not represent a minority group in the traditional sense of the word and therefore should not be regarded in the sense of a class of individuals. Nor are they sufficiently united in their discrimination.[6]

Richard Scotch considers disability activism in an alternative and persuasive way, distinguishing among collective behavior, social movements, and interest groups—with social movements on a continuum between the two. Scotch believes that until the mid-1970s the disability rights movement was a loosely structured grassroots movement. There were few resources available, "leadership by example," and only occasional focusing events that brought activists together.[7] He notes, too, that there are no aggregate data on individual or organizational participants in the disability rights movement, making it difficult to characterize movement adherents or even to say how many people are involved because many people participate in relatively unobservable ways. Most important, however, Scotch believes that a more accurate term is "disability rights movement" rather than simply "disability movement" because there is a critical difference between the two. The disability rights movement has as its goal the empowerment and collective rights of disabled people, whereas other organizations seek to provide services for persons with disabilities (such as rehabilitation, personal attendants, or transportation).[8] For example, Paralyzed Veterans of America works almost exclusively for its specific membership, although it may support broad-based disability issues. In contrast, Disability Rights Advocates is not a membership organization, but it works to assist disabled persons in the judicial arena by representing its clients in litigation.

This distinction is useful because it helps to explain why the disability rights movement has progressed from the early 1970s, when the primary emphasis of the majority of the movement's leadership was on providing benefits for disabled people, and how that changed in the 1980s and 1990s to a focus on discrimination and civil rights.

DISABILITY INTEREST GROUPS

Within the social sciences there is a generally agreed understanding that organized interests are important in shaping public policy because such groups are more attentive to problems and issues than the general public and because they possess the kinds of resources that lead to substantial influence over policy outcomes. There also are differences, however, in the models and approaches that are used to analyze public policymaking. Among early writers, the concept of pluralism probably was the most commonly used model to explain the policymaking process. In its simplest form, pluralism can be regarded as a democratic process that involves bargaining and negotiation among groups and individuals with competing perspectives. Through this process, people and groups pursue their self-interests through government. This approach—espoused by Earl Latham, among others—contends that public policy is the product of group struggles that are a central facet of American political life.[9] Similarly, David Easton proposed his political systems theory to explain the "input-output" process that results from what goes on inside the "black box" of the political system.[10] Easton argued that although the public does provide input, we know little about what happens when that input is "digested" within the political system. Mancur Olson, whose work has been termed by many social scientists the cornerstone of rational self-interest (or social choice or public choice theory, depending on the author) group theory, argues that there is very little incentive for self-interested individuals to join groups. The reason, Olson argues, is that any single member of a group will enjoy only a small fraction of the material benefits accumulated by the entire group. The bulk of the benefits often go to "free riders"—nonmembers who, in effect, garner the benefits of the larger group without having to join or participate in any way.[11]

With regard to American disability policy, no single theory can adequately explain why there has been a significant paradigm shift or why statutes such as the ADA have had mixed success in the attempt to eliminate discrimination against persons with disabilities. One factor is abundantly clear, however: Disability interest groups have played a key role in the policymaking process described in chapter 1, and without their support American disability policy is unlikely to have moved forward during the last decade. Scotch argues that this forward movement is due largely to the result of a change to a rights issue orientation and participation in the identifiable disability rights movement that made individual groups more successful.[12]

Researchers have invested considerable energy in their efforts to explain and identify specific forms of collective action, especially within the context of disability politics. There also have been valuable contributions by those who have chronicled the disability rights movement—from historical perspectives[13] and within the movement itself,[14] as well as within the framework of community integration and deinstitutionalization.[15]

When the issue is the disability rights movement, the typology of groups can become cumbersome and often confusing. One model, developed by James Charlton, differentiates among groups by reviewing their structures and strategies. Charlton breaks disability groups into ten categories:

1. Local self-help groups (small collectives of people providing peer counseling and moral support, often without a specific disability rights agenda because their primary concerns focus on group members)
2. Local advocacy and program centers (primarily, centers for independent living that are nonresidential, not-for-profit organizations that engage in advocacy, service, and public education)
3. Local single-issue advocacy groups (advocacy-oriented organizations concerned with a wide range of issues that often align themselves with larger advocacy groups)
4. Public policy groups (educational centers, institutes, and projects that provide training and conduct research, such as the World Institute on Disability)
5. Single-issue national advocacy groups (organizations that focus on a specific problem, such as accessible transportation or personal attendant services)
6. National membership organizations (groups with local chapters that participate in advocacy and program activities)
7. National coalitions/federations of groups (autonomous organizations that link together and advocate on each other's behalf, such as the National Council on Independent Living)

8. National single-disability organizations (the oldest, most traditional type of disability group, often apolitical and focused on a particular type of disability, such as blindness)
9. Regional organizations (federations of groups that are not national in scope, often organized on a state level)
10. International organizations (groups such as Mobility International, which has a global focus).[16]

This typology of organizations is part of the assumption that a disability rights social movement exists in the United States. Although the literature of social movements chronicles groups that focus on a wide range of issues, from the environment to civil rights to nuclear weapons, there is some consensus about their common characteristics. Among those characteristics are the following:

- They seek to connect the personal (or cultural) and political realms.
- They attempt to raise psychological issues that often have been submerged or ignored.[17]
- They have a cohesiveness that focuses on moral justness and ethical issues.

Disability policy is an outgrowth of a social movement for civil rights for disabled people. Although it stems from a wide spectrum of interest groups, it also has been affected by the political environment of the policy process described in greater detail in chapter 3.

BERKELEY AND THE INDEPENDENT LIVING MOVEMENT

The Center for Independent Living (CIL) movement began in the 1960s, sparked by disabled students at the University of California, Berkeley, who lived at Cowell Hospital, the university's infirmary. The housing program was managed by the California Department of Rehabilitation as a medically based facility for severely disabled students. Among those living at

Cowell was Ed Roberts, a respiratory quadriplegic who became inspired by the political and social activism that accompanied the free speech, civil rights, and feminist movements sweeping across college campuses. Roberts and several other residents established The Rolling Quads, a group of students who protested the often arbitrary requirements placed on their lives by the department's counselors. Roberts and his cohort realized that because they were segregated from the rest of the community by being housed at Cowell, they were missing out on traditional college life and still faced numerous barriers, architectural and otherwise, that defined the university experience.

Roberts went to Washington, D.C., in 1969 and met with officials at the U.S. Department of Health, Education, and Welfare (HEW), including Jean Wirth, who had established a support program for minority students. Roberts was asked to design a program for disabled students that would later become the Physically Disabled Students Program. At its core was the belief that the best way to determine what disabled students needed was to involve them in the decision-making process, developing a comprehensive program that included provisions for personal assistance services, and integrating disabled students into mainstream university life. HEW began funding for the program in July 1970, and although it was originally intended to serve University of California students, nonstudents began to apply for assistance as well. Realizing that there was a need for a full-service program that was community based and dedicated to deinstitutionalization, Berkeley's CIL was opened with Ed Roberts as its first executive director and a $50,000 grant from the Rehabilitation Services Administration.

Boston and Berkeley were the first cities to establish community-based independent living centers, although Berkeley usually is given credit for being the birthplace of the concept because the Boston center began to offer transitional housing and attendant care in 1974.[18] The CIL's mission varied somewhat during the 1970s. Most of its supporters agreed that the strongest need was for an advocacy program for the disabled community, rather than a social services center. As a part of that philosophy, the CIL provided the impetus for the founding of the Disability Law Resource Center (now called the Disability Rights Education and Defense Fund). The CIL movement also provided the political training ground for many of the disability rights activists who would move on to lobby for other federal policies.[19]

"THE SPLINTERED UNIVERSE"

One of the slogans often associated with disability activism is "Nothing About Us Without Us"—a phrase that has parallel significance with "Power to the People" in the civil rights movement and, for many in the women's liberation movement, "Our Bodies, Ourselves." Ed Roberts often is quoted as having said, "If we have learned one thing from the civil rights movement in the [United States], it's that when others speak for you, you lose."[20] Activist/author James Charlton uses the slogan to capture the essence of the changing paradigm of disability rights. "[It] requires people with disabilities to recognize their need to control and take responsibility for their own lives. It also forces political-economic and cultural systems to incorporate people with disabilities into the decision-making process and to recognize that the experiential knowledge of these people is pivotal in making decisions that affect their lives."[21]

The successes and failures of American disability policy often can be tied to the fact that disabled people do not speak with one voice. In calling the disability rights movement a "splintered universe," writer Joseph Shapiro notes, "There are hundreds of different disabilities, and each group tended to see its issues in relation to its specific disability. There were groups for people with head injuries, different groups for blind people, and still others for cancer survivors or those with diabetes, arthritis, learning disabilities, and mental illness, all fighting for specific programs, funding, and laws to address the needs of members of their own group."[22]

Shapiro goes on to cite examples of the cross-cutting priorities of various groups. Wheelchair users, he notes, fought for curb cuts that would allow them access to sidewalks, but blind people with canes, who tapped curbs for a sense of location, often wanted the curbs left untouched. Even organizations representing the same type of disability clashed among themselves. The National Federation for the Blind (NFB), for example, refused to add its support to the ADA, which had the endorsement of the American Council of the Blind. The NFB—perhaps more militant in its approach than other groups—argues that blind people do not need any special type of help, lest they be considered inferior to those who are not blind.

COALITION BUILDING AND CROSS-DISABILITY ACTIVISM

The ADA's supporters knew from the very beginning that the disabled rights movement's fragmentation would sound a death knell for passage of the ADA. Instead, they managed to build a coalition of national and local groups that had never been brought together before, as illustrated in Box 4.1.

Although some of the coalition building was deliberate, at other times it was almost serendipitous. The March 1990 Wheels of Justice March, for example, just happened to take place at the same time that the National Rehabilitation Association (NRA) was holding its legislative convention in Washington, D.C. Members of the group, founded in 1920, frequently had been criticized by disability activists who felt that rehabilitation professionals were not doing enough for their clients and that many persons with disabilities were falling through the cracks of the health care system. Yet members of the NRA canceled several morning sessions of their conference so they could join the protest in front of the White House.

Of particular importance in the coalition-building process was the involvement of gay rights activists, who fought to have people with AIDS or those who are HIV-positive included under the protection of the ADA. The initial argument was that both were chronic illnesses, no different from tuberculosis or cancer; therefore, persons with these conditions ought to be covered by the ADA as well. The issue was especially critical for people who had been discriminated against in the workplace when the nature of their illness was discovered or voluntarily disclosed.[23]

BOX 4.1

Leading Organizations Advocating on Behalf of the ADA (1988–1990)

AIDS Action Council
AIDS National InterFaith Network
American Civil Liberties Foundation
American Foundation for the Blind
Americans Disabled for Accessible Public Transit
Association for Education and Rehabilitation of the Blind and Visually
   Handicapped
Association for Retarded Citizens
Consortium for Citizens with Disabilities
Disability Rights Education and Defense Fund
Dole Foundation
Eastern Paralyzed Veterans of America
Epilepsy Foundation of America
Human Rights Campaign Fund
Institute for Rehabilitation and Research
Leadership Conference on Civil Rights
Legal Action Center
Mental Health Law Project
National Association of Developmental Disabilities Councils
National Association of Protection and Advocacy Systems
National Center for Law and the Deaf
National Council of Independent Living
National Council on Disability
National Disability Action Center
National Easter Seals Society
National Organization Responding to AIDS
Paralyzed Veterans of America
President's Committee on Employment of People with Disabilities
Spina Bifida Association of America
United Cerebral Palsy Association

Source: Adapted from Disability Rights Education and Defense Fund,
ADA Gala, February 1, 1992.

Many of the ADA's supporters also realized that unlike their own movement, the gay rights lobby was much more cohesive and held considerable
political and financial clout. Adding their numbers and political expertise to the disability movement was a major bonus for many disability
rights activists. Members of Congress and some activist groups were not
so sure, however, given the homophobia that still characterized representatives from conservative districts. Rural Texas Representative Ralph Hall,
for instance, is quoted as telling the members of the NRA that he didn't
"want to hand out anything more to those damn homosexuals." His views,
he said, were a reflection of his constituents' values and a result of the hundreds of letters he had received from fundamentalist churches urging him
to oppose the ADA.[24]

Some of the organizations with a cross-disability focus, such as the
United Parent Syndicate on Disabilities are part of the larger family advocacy movements. The addition of groups advocating for children was a
major boost for the ADA's supporters because many of the parents had been
active in the earlier legislative struggles to provide educational opportunities for children. The earliest parents' movement had begun in the 1930s,
especially among the families of children with mental retardation and cerebral palsy. After World War II, the groups included the National Alliance
for the Mentally Ill, the National Association of Retarded Children (now
called the Arc), and the Federation for Children with Special Needs.

The parent groups also had the advantages of larger budgets and a membership structure that had been developed over decades. Their issues
involved not only the entire spectrum of types of disabilities but other
related issues, such as health care reform and adaptive technology. The
more radical of the groups, such as Mothers From Hell, gave additional
credibility to the more mainstream organizations.[25]

Despite the fact that often-competing groups came together to support
the ADA, years of political differences and strategies have become a critical mass of activism only recently. As Charlton notes, although the disability rights movement continues to grow, "it is still small and its 'Let's all
get together' ideological center of gravity is soft and shallow."[26]

DEMONSTRATIONS AND PROTESTS

The literature of social movements finds that, as a general rule, protests are a very short-lived form of collective association. They must begin with a clearly defined grievance that involves people who are less powerful or powerless, and they must use means that are generally disruptive against a clearly defined target.[27] Some will have short-term success (such as the ouster of Rinser as president of Gallaudet), as well as longer-term achievements (such as legitimization of a deaf culture movement).

In the early 1970s one of the preeminent protest organizations was Disabled in Action (DIA), a group originally formed to increase opportunities for disabled persons to join in the mainstream of societal life. The group had been established by Judy Heumann, a post-polio paraplegic who had been denied teaching certification after her graduation from Long Island University. She filed a highly publicized lawsuit that brought together individuals with a broad range of disabilities, forming a core of about eighty supporters (most of whom lived on the east coast). Their demonstrations focused on inaccessible public buildings, the Jerry Lewis telethon, discriminatory stereotypes, and media coverage of disability issues. Among their most visible protests was one against the New York reelection headquarters of Richard Nixon in 1972 after the president had vetoed the Rehabilitation Act, as well as a subsequent protest in Washington, D.C., when he vetoed a similar bill a second time.[28]

Within the disability rights movement, the most visible protest organization today is American Disabled for Accessible Public Transit (ADAPT).[29] In Mary Johnson and Barry Shaw's historical account of the fight for accessible transportation, *To Ride the Public's Buses: The Fight that Built a Movement,*[30] the story begins in 1973 with Metropolitan Area Disabled (MAD), a group of sixty nursing home residents in Denver. The group met regularly, and its members worked in cooperation with Atlantis Community—another group that provided attendant services for people who were no longer living in the nursing home. Atlantis attorneys sued the Denver Regional Transportation District in 1977, seeking accessible transportation beyond the city's dozen minibuses (called paratransit). Shortly after the group lost in court in June 1978, wheelchair activists and supporters surrounded two municipal buses, keeping them out of service to focus attention on the fact that the buses were not accessible to people who could not climb steps. For the next year and a half, the group disrupted meetings of the transit district's board, occupied offices, and initiated a ballot measure that called for the board to be elected by the public. By 1983 the transit district had not only ordered new accessible buses but made a commitment that there would be lifts on all of the vehicles on its routes. In the process, the rapid transit district changed directors after a newly hired director ordered buses that were not accessible. The protestors chained themselves in the district's offices, then worked with other organizations to elect board members who were committed to accessibility. The director was fired, and the city has continued to maintain its reputation for having an accessible public transit system for all of its citizens.[31]

Also in 1983, ADAPT—founded by Wade Blank, a minister and political activist who learned political organizing from the civil rights movement—focused on the annual meeting of the American Public Transit Association (APTA), which was scheduled for October in Denver. APTA became the target of yearly protests as demonstrators attempted to block access to the group's convention and held candlelight vigils, marches, and other actions designed to disrupt the conferences.[32]

When the ADA came under congressional scrutiny in 1989, many of ADAPT's leaders shifted their attention to Washington. Among their most successful protests was the March 1990 Wheels of Justice March, bringing an estimated 1,000 demonstrators to the Capitol. On March 12, 1989, nearly 100 wheelchair users participated in a widely publicized "crawl-up" on the steps of the Capitol building. The following day, ADAPT took over the Capitol rotunda; dozens of demonstrators were arrested. The images on the nightly news were compelling, and some observers believe that ADAPT's more militant stance on the ADA helped push the legislation through Congress at a critical time in its development.

Some ADA advocates, however, believed that the Capitol protests were counterproductive because they sent a mixed message to the American public and legislators. The news coverage of paraplegics on their hands and knees trying to crawl the eighty-three steps up the front of the Capitol simply reinforced old stereotypes and images that many protestors had fought to eliminate. More moderate supporters, such as Senator Bob Dole of Kansas, walked past the demonstration and said, "This doesn't help us any"—a remark echoed by Randy Jennings, one of the rehabilitation association's leaders.[33]

Today, ADAPT has an estimated 5,000 members in twenty-nine states. The group's agenda has broadened, but protest and civil disobedience continue to be the primary modus operandi. In 1998 the group held a four-day protest in Washington, D.C., that included a takeover of the Democratic and Republican headquarters, as well as the Department of Health and Human Services main administrative center. The demonstrations, which involved about 700 ADAPT members, were part of the group's Campaign for REAL Choice on the eve of the 1998 elections. According to an ADAPT press release, the action campaign "is about getting a national system of home and community-based attendant services"; the release noted that despite the ADA's "most integrated setting mandate," more than three-fourths of all Medicaid long-term care dollars go to institutional care.[34]

ADAPT continues to make accessible transportation one of its primary goals—as Greyhound Bus Lines found out in 1998. The company, which had come under considerable pressure from disabled activists for its failure to install permanent ramps to its fleet of buses in violation of the ADA, faced off against protestors in thirty-five cities on January 15, 1998. Using their bodies and wheelchairs as roadblocks, ADAPT members held hour-long demonstrations that delayed departing buses throughout the United States. One San Francisco resident remarked as he was being arrested, "We're just glad to see that the bus to take us to jail is accessible. We wish Greyhound was, as well."[35]

Researchers have identified several factors that have made demonstrations and protests an important element of social activism within the disability rights movement:

1. *A supportive political and cultural climate.* Neil Smelser argues that this is a basic precondition for the success of any type of collective action. Protests must be seen as an acceptable strategy for social change within the political environment of the time. In the case of the disability community, activists have been able to piggyback on several decades of protests—from the civil rights movement during the 1950s and 1960s to a residue of support from people who had engaged in student protests during the 1960s and 1970s. Campuses had become a natural setting for student activism by the time the Gallaudet DPN protest began, and the steps of the Capitol in Washington, D.C., have become the photo-op *du jour* for any group seeking media attention.

Nonviolent protests and mass confrontations have become an acceptable form of collective behavior, measured by political scientists as part of a range of types of political participation (along with voting and contributing to a political candidate). The public—with a few exceptions, such as the World Trade Organization demonstrations in Seattle in 2000—generally is tolerant of such displays of opinion, and the strategy itself is almost expected. Tilly notes that groups are more likely to use tactics with which they are familiar, rather than innovative ones, and disabled rights activists rarely have deviated from this model.[36]

2. *The type of issue.* Not all protests are successful, of course, and those of the disability rights movement are no exception. Biklen cites two factors that contribute to a group's success: The issue must be interesting and morally persuasive.[37] Many researchers who have chronicled the development of disability policy believe that one of the successful devices used by group leaders was to frame the issue as one of civil rights rather than disability rights. In the Gallaudet protest, demonstrators carried a banner to the Capitol that read, "I have a dream"—linking their march to the 1963 gathering at which Martin Luther King, Jr., made his famous speech.

Similarly, during the fight for passage of the ADA, leaders were careful to note that they were not seeking any form of "special" rights for persons with disabilities; instead, they wanted the extension of basic civil rights to PWDs. The strategy, according to Christiansen and Barnartt, was to gain support for their demands from the general public. "Wittingly or unwittingly, the protesters' perspective encouraged more sympathy and support for their demands than they might have received if they had framed the issue in a different way."[38] In addition, the protestors framed the issue in limited terms. They were very explicit in their demands that the president of Gallaudet be a deaf person; there was no attempt made to expand their demonstration outside the campus walls.

One of the factors that made ADAPT so successful in the beginning was its singular focus on accessible transportation. Initially, ADAPT's goal was to make sure that all municipal transit bus systems were equipped with wheelchair lifts—providing mobility that was synonymous with freedom and equality. As Atlanta ADAPT activist Mark Johnson said, "Black people fought for the right to ride in the front of the bus. We're fighting for the right to get on the bus."[39] The issue was easily understood by the public, and most members agreed to use nonviolent civil disobedience as a protest strategy. The group's simple slogan, "We will ride!" stood out from the complex issues surrounding the removal of architectural and programmatic barriers.

3. *Mobilization and cohesiveness.* After the 1973 protests by Disabled in Action, leaders realized that they needed to change their image from one of "rabble-rousing kids" to that of a more cohesive group that reached out to other disability organizations. As one participant noted, "We had to not only get together in order to agree upon what we could support, but also because it would give us a much louder stronger voice."[40] That voice became the American Coalition of Citizens with Disabilities, which represented the interests of about sixty-five national and local affiliated organizations and operated out of the New York Mayor's Office for the Handicapped. The coalition was able not only to build bridges among the various groups who were members but also to establish a presence in Washington to lobby members of Congress.

One factor that helped to mobilize the students at Gallaudet was the ability of the protest leaders to recruit other students because they were in close proximity on the campus. Although it has been reported that, at least initially, students felt they had little to gain, a sense of cohesiveness began to develop when the issue was reframed as "an end to oppression by hearing people." At that point, even those who cared little about the university president jumped on the bandwagon because they could identify with others who could not hear.[41] Cohesive groups, Miller has argued, are "glued" together—which increases their chances of success.[42] Along with the sense of group cohesiveness was the sense of "protest euphoria" that developed. A demonstration produces a type of political high that is accentuated by factors that are hard to quantify: the pulsating beat of drums, chants (or, in the case of Gallaudet, mass signing), spring weather, a release from school examinations, the presence of the media. As during the student protests against the Vietnam war in the late 1960s, in some ways being part of a student demonstration is a rite of college passage. It draws in even those who would otherwise be marginalized or reluctant to participate.

4. *Support and resources.* Early on, it was clear to advocates who were building the disability rights movement that they needed more than just their own members' support to make any real progress. As Scotch notes, many of the early activists had found jobs within the Washington establishment, with individual members of Congress and as staffers on committees and within federal agencies. These individuals, who knew how to get inside Washington's halls of power, helped advocates get support from the government. Sometimes this support took the form of grants; at other times it simply meant gaining entrance to meet with a member of Congress. These strategies, however, helped disability rights advocates gain acceptability and created an atmosphere of receptiveness that helped the broader movement.[43]

Gallaudet alumni provided resources for the 1988 protest, as did the university's faculty. The Washington, D.C., deaf community—many of whom are Gallaudet graduates—joined in support, as did students at other residential deaf schools. There was a large donation from a labor union, as well as support from others with physical disabilities, local church and community groups, and hearing students at other Washington-area colleges.

LITIGATION

Chapter 1 briefly identifies the role of the courts in shaping policy, and it is important to recognize that litigation has become an important tool in the disability rights movement, before and after the passage of the ADA.

"When all else fails, sue the bastards," is the claim of one disability rights attorney as he describes his attempt to change disability policy through litigation. For many advocates, recourse to the courts, especially as an individual plaintiff, is the final step on a very long and costly road. For disabled plaintiffs, the action is made even more difficult by the lack of accessible facilities to even begin the process of litigation, communication problems, and confusion over the law. The ADA, many observers believe, is still too "young" to have developed a solid base of case law (an issue discussed in more depth in chapter 6). As a result, litigation by individuals sometimes is less likely to succeed than cases brought as class actions by multiple plaintiffs.

One of the exceptions occurred in 1997 when a thirty-two-year-old deaf student at Gallaudet was awarded $1,500 by a U.S. District Court jury. The student tried to place an order at a drive-through window of a McDonald's restaurant by writing his order on a piece of paper. His order initially was refused, and the plaintiff was told to park and go inside the restaurant. When he refused, backing up a line of cars, he was given the wrong order and his complaints brought a request for him to leave the premises. He did not leave and was arrested by an off-duty police officer; eventually he sued the company for emotional distress. The judge, ruling on additional issues, said the franchise discriminated against deaf people and those with hearing impairments and ordered McDonald's to better train its employees to accommodate deaf customers.[44]

Lest this case sound like a happy ending to an unhappy story, however, it also should be noted that the case took nineteen months to wend its way through the federal court system, and the resulting monetary award was hardly a litigant's dream come true. The plaintiff testified that "he wished he had never been born," and money clearly was not the overriding factor in his decision to sue McDonald's.

One of the factors that has helped disabled litigants has been the growth of state protection and advocacy (P&A) organizations. Their influence stems from a variety of factors. In 1975 the Developmentally Disabled Assistance and Bill of Rights Act[45] gave the federal and state governments the right to withhold funds from institutions that did not meet minimum standards of care, partially as a result of investigations of abuse at various state facilities such as Willowbrook in New York. As part of its enforcement mechanism, the statute also required the governor of each state to designate an agency (public or private) to provide protection and advocacy services.

Several additions and changes have been made since the law was passed, although the system remains relatively unchanged. Clients of vocational rehabilitation programs were added to the protective network in 1984 under amendments to the Rehabilitation Act.[46] In 1986 the Protection and Advocacy for Mentally Ill Individuals Act gave additional support through funding and technical assistance from the National Center for Mental Health Services.[47] In 1988 the Technology Related Assistance for Individuals with Disabilities Act provided P&A assistance to help families and people with disabilities gain access to assistive technology. In 1994 the P&A system was expanded again to cover Native Americans. Once established, such programs were eager to take on ADA compliance cases. In Texas, for example, Advocacy, Inc. initially filed fifty-three lawsuits against health care providers, convenience stores, attorneys' offices, retail stores, theaters, restaurants, banks, and day care centers.[48] Although litigation has been important to some individual complainants, the ADA has brought a trend toward more class-action lawsuits (a strategy that is discussed in depth in chapter 6).

The federal government administers P&A programs through the U.S. Department of Health and Human Services and the U.S. Department of

Education's Rehabilitation Services Administration. The National Association of Protection and Advocacy Systems serves as the national coordinating body and as a membership organization for the various state programs.

It can be argued that the strategies and concerns of the contemporary disability rights movement have changed little from its historical roots— the League of the Physically Handicapped. San Francisco State University historian Paul Longmore and researcher David Goldberger chronicle the group's protest against disability-related job discrimination at New York City's Emergency Relief Bureau in 1935. Six people staged a sit-in, demanding to see the agency's director, and vowed that they would occupy the office until he arrived or until "Hell freezes over." At the time, the movement consisted primarily of individuals who were polio survivors or people with other chronic illnesses such as cerebral palsy; there were no League members who used wheelchairs, or were blind or deaf. They redefined themselves, Longmore and Goldberger write, as "handicapped." "Their activism sought to alter public understanding of disabilities, shifting the focus from coping with impairment to managing identity, from experiencing polio to engaging in politics."[49]

Officials tried to isolate the protestors by denying them food, but more supporters—most of them not handicapped—picketed and organized mass demonstrations. Some of the protestors were arrested, brought before a judge who seemed not to know what to do with "the Communist cripples," and lambasted by the press. Yet the month-long demonstrations not only gained the group public attention but also gave them sufficient funds to open an office and organize as the League of the Physically Handicapped, which focuses on job discrimination.[50]

There are several differences between the League's mission and the disability movement today. The League's members advocated incremental reform rather than the kinds of systemic change the ADA exemplifies. In the League's day, disability leaders borrowed from the labor and leftist groups; after World War II, disability groups looked to the civil rights and feminist movements to identify potential strategies. During the Depression years, the League sought employment as a way of providing economic security for their members. Now, organizations representing persons with disabilities are split between those offering specific services and support (often to individuals with a specific disability) and those focusing on cross-disability issues and political advocacy. The young adults with disabilities who met at a New York recreation center or in basement clubs generally shared a common ethnic, religious, and socioeconomic background; now, disability activists represent the heterogeneity of disability itself.

What remains to be seen is whether the groups and individuals who pressed the agenda of the ADA will suffer the same fate as that of the League. Longmore and Goldberger note that the League disbanded around 1938 as a result of internal disputes and its successes in gaining employment. It never sought to change societal attitudes, reform the social welfare system, or form a broader coalition for political purposes. "The League failed to establish an institutional base upon which to build further activism by physically handicapped people. . . . There was no direct line of descent, no institutional or even individual continuity, from the league to any later activist organization."[51]

The remaining chapters of this book explore how those differences in focus and mission affected not only the passage of the ADA but its implementation and resulting policies. By comparing the old with the new, it is possible to draw some conclusions about changing paradigms first outlined in the Introduction and developed further in chapter 8.

CHAPTER 5

The ADA and the Vision of Equality

If it were possible to identify any single individual who was most responsible for the passage of the 1990 Americans with Disabilities Act, most activists probably would name Justin Dart, Jr. Dart, who was born in 1930, came from a wealthy Chicago family; he contracted polio in 1948, prior to entering the University of Houston. His undergraduate degree was in history and education, but the university's officials refused to give him a teaching certificate because of his disability. He went on to organize the first student group opposing racism at the then-segregated university and in 1954 earned his master's degree in history.

Dart's entrepreneurial skills helped him found three successful Japanese corporations, and he traveled widely throughout the Far East, visiting institutions for the disabled. In 1967 he gave up his corporate life for one devoted to the rights of disabled persons, working tirelessly in Texas and, later on, in Washington, D.C., as a member of various state and federal disability commissions. During the Reagan administration, he refused to support the president's efforts to revise the 1973 Rehabilitation Act, and in 1993 he quit his position on the President's Committee on Employment of People with Disabilities—a position he had held since his nomination by President George Bush in 1989.

Dart's personal commitment to disability rights is best represented by his involvement in the battle for the ADA—more accurately explained as the culmination of years of activism that had previously focused on Section 504 of the Rehabilitation Act. Dart argued with many of his colleagues within the disability community who felt that the 1973 law had marked the end of contemporary civil rights struggles. He disagreed, writing, "Around 1980 it became clear to me that we would never overcome the barriers to mainstream participation until the message of our full humanity was communicated into the consciousness and political process of America by a strong, highly visible, comprehensive civil rights law. It was equally clear that no meaningful mandate for equality could be passed or implemented until our tiny, fragmented disability community movement united, expanded, and matured in the political process."[1]

President Bush signed the ADA into law on July 26, 1990, with Dart among those on the dais. Dart subsequently served as a donor to disability organizations across the United States and was a principal organizer for numerous ADA anniversary events. With other activists, he founded Justice For All to defend congressional attempts to weaken the ADA, and he helped found the American Association of People with Disabilities in 1995. He received the Presidential Medal of Freedom in 1998.

Speaking at a meeting in Alexandria, Virginia, in 2000—just after the tenth anniversary celebration of the ADA's passage—Dart commented that he believed that "the ADA has been more successful than anyone expected." He also warned, however, that the next decade should focus on "keeping the promise of the ADA. All we have dreamed is possible. All we have gained is at risk [in the 2000 election]."[2] Dart was one of the most beloved members of the disability community, serving as both a leader and an inspirational force for the movement. With his ever-present hat perched precariously on his head, his strong voice resonated out of proportion to those who mistakenly perceived that he was too old or too weak to lead. "I love you," he unabashedly told his audience—who would respond, "We love you, too!"

Dart died at his home in Washington, D.C., on June 21, 2002, after having struggled with the complications of post-polio syndrome and congestive heart failure. Disability rights activists around the world mourned his pass-

ing with praise that Dart would have deflected. He routinely cited others'
accomplishments instead of his own, and it was his wish that any service or
commemoration be used to celebrate the movement—and as an opportunity to recommit to what he called "the revolution of empowerment."

The accolades from others speak to the heart of the old soldier, as Dart
called himself. Words and phrases sped lightning-quick across the Internet
as word of his death traveled. Most common were those who called Dart
"a hero," "courageous," "a beacon in the disability rights movement," and
"an inspiring leader." In his last written words, Dart called for solidarity
among those who love justice, saying, "Let my final actions thunder of
love, solidarity, protest—of empowerment."[3]

This chapter analyzes the events and actors in what Joseph Shapiro calls
"a hidden army for civil rights" that coalesced sufficiently to capture political interest just long enough to convince Congress and President George
Bush to enact the ADA. Shapiro, who has published one of the most thor-
ough chronicles of the disability rights movement, notes that although
"passage of the ADA was an earthshaking event for disabled people . . . nondisabled Americans still had little understanding that this group now
demanded rights, not pity."[4]

This perspective is one of the factors that makes the statute valuable as
a case study because it heralded the last of the nation's twentieth-century
civil rights laws.

This chapter also reviews the ways in which members of the silent army
joined together throughout the legislative process that culminated with the
signing of the ADA. It notes efforts at coalition building, inclusion of
political leaders who supported the campaign, questions raised over what
types of disabilities ought to be covered by the law, and opposition
mounted to defeat it.

DEVELOPING A NATIONAL POLICY: EARLY INITIATIVES

Forty years prior to the passage of the ADA, Congress enacted several disability discrimination laws (see Box 5.1). These laws represent a pattern

BOX 5.1

Major Disability Legislation Enacted Prior to Passage of 1990 Americans with Disabilities Act

1948	Act of June 10, 1948
1965	Rehabilitation Act Amendments (Title V)
1968	Architectural Barriers Act
1970	Developmental Disabilities Services and Facilities Construction Amendments
	Urban Mass Transportation Assistance Act
1973	Rehabilitation Act
1975	Education of All Handicapped Children Act
	Developmental Disabilities Assistance and Bill of Rights Act
1978	Rehabilitation Act Amendments
1980	Civil Rights of Institutionalized Persons Act
1982	Telephone Communications for the Disabled Act
1984	Voting Accessibility for the Elderly And Handicapped Act
1986	Air Carrier Access Act
	Protection and Advocacy for Mentally Ill Individuals Act
	Rehabilitation Act Amendments
1988	Fair Housing Amendments Act

of incremental decision making that characterizes American disability policy. The early initiatives are important because they formed the legal basis for the ADA, but they never had the impact on civil rights that the ADA eventually did.

The first step in the development of what was to become the ADA was to come to consensus about what a new civil rights law ought to include. The process began in 1982 when the National Council on the Handicapped (NCH—later renamed the National Council on Disability, or NCD) directed Justin Dart to gather recommendations for a comprehensive disability policy. A national campaign encouraged people with disabilities to write "discrimination diaries" that documented instances in which they had faced barriers to access or other forms of discrimination so that it would become clear that such discrimination often was a daily facet of life. After holding public hearings throughout the country, the council developed a policy document that recommended a separate civil rights law that recognized the distinctive nature of discrimination against disabled people. The NCD—an independent federal agency whose members were appointed by President Reagan—produced a 1986 report to the president and Congress, *Toward Independence,*[5] and a follow-up report, *On the Threshold of Independence,*[6] that became the basis for legislation introduced in 1988 in the 100th Congress by Connecticut Senator Lowell Weicker. The first draft of the legislation had been developed by the NCD's counsel, Robert L. Burgdorf, Jr., whose upper right arm was paralyzed as a result of the polio he contracted the same year as Dart. Burgdorf's version of a disability rights law was virtually ignored by Congress and the press. Some advocates believe the 1988 bill was sabotaged by White House Chief of Staff John Sununu, who argued with Attorney General Dick Thornburgh over the accessibility standards in the proposal, as well as the potential damages that could be levied on small businesses.[7]

A year later, a revised bill was written by Bobby Silverstein, director of the Senate Subcommittee on the Handicapped; the bill was reintroduced into the 101st Congress by Iowa senator Tom Harkin and California representative Tony Coelho, among others. In September 1988, Congress held joint hearings where hundreds of witnesses testified about the injustices they faced and the pervasiveness of stereotypes and prejudice. (The actual process of legislative deliberation is outlined in more detail later in this chapter.)

What makes the ADA an important case study for many people, however, is the fact that the statute is not just one more example of how a bill becomes a law. The story of the ADA could have followed a very predictable process of introduction, debate, vote, and signing that often is taught in school classrooms. Instead, this book argues that the ADA was enacted as a result of several specific, identifiable factors that, at another time, might have failed. It passed because the policy window opened for a steadily growing, cohesive coalition of groups that were able to take advantage of their political support within Congress when the political environment was favorable to their interests. The remainder of this chapter chronicles how this happened.

OPENING THE POLICY WINDOW

John Kingdon describes the policy window as "an opportunity for advocates of proposals to push their pet solutions or to push attention to their special problems."[8] He notes that sometimes advocates "lie in wait and around government with their solutions at hand, waiting for problems to float by to which they can attach their solutions, waiting for a development in the political stream they can use to their advantage. Sometimes, the window opens quite predictably. . . . At other times, it happens quite unpredictably."[9]

Kingdon goes on to explain that the policy window's openings and closings can be thought of as a queue of items waiting their turn on a decision agenda. "Somehow, the items must be ordered in the queue. The opening of a window often establishes the priority in the queue. Participants move some items ahead of others, essentially because they believe the proposals stand a decent chance of enactment."[10]

Supporters of an issue often must wait their turn as other issues take precedence or as the political environment changes. For disability rights activists, the policy window opened slightly during the administration of Jimmy Carter when the president required that all new transit systems and newly acquired buses be wheelchair accessible. Just as the window appeared to open a crack or two, however, it closed as the president focused on foreign policy issues. Domestic concerns took a back seat to the Iran hostage crisis, oil shortages, and the political rise of Ronald Reagan. Once elected, Reagan rescinded Carter's order on accessible transit, closing the policy window for much of his two terms as president.

Researcher Sara Watson notes that the 1980s were marked by political hostility and public indifference. For eight years the Reagan administration reduced funding for services for the disabled and made an attempt to roll back some of the previous administrations' antidiscrimination efforts. At the same time, disability issues were not on the public's radar screen or anyone's political agenda. "No public opinion poll had highlighted disability discrimination as a major issue; no new publication had captured the public's attention; no crisis had emerged to spur legislators to action; no data had suddenly emerged to indicate a dramatic increase in problematic behavior; and no media expose had taken place."[11] The reason the policy window opened for the ADA in the late 1980s can be found partially in the policy environment of the time.

POLICY ENVIRONMENT

Although it is generally agreed that the ADA was an important extension of Section 504 of the 1973 Rehabilitation Act (see chapter 2), several other factors can be considered critical to the opening of the policy window for the ADA's supporters. Arlene Mayerson, an advocate who is known for her perspectives on the disability rights movement in her role as an attorney with the Disability Rights Education and Defense Fund, believes that supporters faced an extremely hostile policy environment at the time.[12] What came to be known as the "regulatory reform" movement had taken place under three presidents: Nixon, Ford, and Carter. During the 1970s, deregulation was targeted at two areas: economic regulation that controlled entry into the regulated field (such as banking and public utilities) and "the new regulation," which included statutes and agencies relating to the environment, safety, and health.[13]

One of the most crucial fights was the disability rights movement's battle to defend Section 504's regulations from the onslaught of the Reagan administration. As one of his initial official acts, Reagan established the Task Force on Regulatory Relief, part of his campaign promise to "get the government off the people's backs." The task force, headed by Vice President George Bush, was charged with bringing deregulation to as many policy areas as possible—especially policies that were considered burdensome to businesses. Many of the targets of deregulation were related to the flurry of environmental protection statutes that had been passed during the 1970s, including the 1977 Clean Air Act and amendments to clean water legislation. Reagan's charge to the task force was to continue the process of deregulation initiated by his predecessors; Bush moved quickly to tackle his new responsibilities. Among the targets of the task force were the Section 504 regulations.[14]

A second major factor that mobilized disability rights activists during the 1980s was a series of U.S. Supreme Court decisions that had the effect of reducing protections against discrimination. One of the most important cases was the decision in *Grove City College v. Bell*, 465 U.S. 555 (1984), which restricted the reach of prior statutes that prohibited recipients of federal funds from discriminating against individuals on the basis of race, ethnic origin, sex, or disability. The case affected the four major civil rights statutes that had been passed since 1964, including Section 504 of the Rehabilitation Act. The case involved a college student who brought suit under Title IX of the Education Amendments of 1972, arguing that she had been discriminated against by a department of her college on the basis of her gender. The Supreme Court ruled against her, however, deciding that regardless of whether discrimination had actually occurred, the department itself had not received any federal funds, thereby voiding any protection against discrimination. Even though the case involved gender discrimination, by extension it also voided protection for people with disabilities.

A second 1984 case further alarmed advocates who believed their civil rights protections had a firm legal basis. In *Jacobson v. Delta Airlines*, 742 F. 2d 1202 (1984), a suit was brought against the airline's policy of requiring disabled passengers to sign a statement before boarding in which they agreed to be removed from the plane at any time for unspecified reasons. The case was similar to *Grove City* because the airline also received federal funding. In a third case, *Salve Regina College v. Russell*, 501 U.S. 1203 (1991), a Section 504 complaint by a former teacher against a nursing school was dismissed when the court ruled that the school had received federal funds only through financial aid for its students, thus voiding the civil rights protections for faculty.

Another important case, *Consolidated Rail Corporation v. Darrone*, 465 U.S. 624 (1984), took on the issue of whether employment was covered by the antidiscrimination provisions of Section 504. Several disability rights groups filed *amicus curiae* briefs in the case that documented the types of discrimination faced by disabled workers. In its ruling in favor of the defendant employee, the Supreme Court reaffirmed the protections afforded employees by the Rehabilitation Act.

LEGISLATIVE BUILDING BLOCKS

Throughout the 1980s, advocates worked on several fronts to build what have been called "legislative building blocks" that led to the passage of the ADA.[15] Although statutes such as the Architectural Barriers Act of 1968[16] and the 1975 Developmentally Disabled Assistance and Bill of Rights Act[17] had covered some groups of disabled persons, as had the 1980 Civil Rights of Institutionalized Persons Act,[18] they did not provide the type of broad protection against discrimination sought by the majority of disability right activists.

To blunt the effect of decisions that had narrowed protection under Section 504, a coalition of civil rights groups joined together in the 1980s to seek legislative redress for the damage done by an indifferent, if not hostile, Supreme Court. One of the most important of these incremental changes was the coalition's support of what would become the Civil Rights Restoration Act, first introduced into Congress in February 1985. Later the bill was substantially rewritten, and after overturning President Reagan's veto, Congress enacted the new statute in March 1988.[19] The law was much more specific in defining previously vague provisions in civil rights laws related to what constituted federal funding.

Advocates also managed to create a more positive environment for disability issues in Congress by using the legislative process to overturn other court cases that had narrowed discrimination protection. With the Air

Carriers Access Act of 1986 (49 U.S.C. app. 1374(c)), which reinstated the application of antidiscrimination protections to airline passengers, the movement's leaders were successful in overturning *U.S. Department of Transportation v. Paralyzed Veterans of America,* 477 U.S. 597 (1986). Similarly, the Civil Rights and Remedies Equalization Act of 1986 (42 U.S.C. 2000d-7) gave disabled persons the right to sue states for violations of Section 504, overturning the ruling in *Atascadero State Hospital v. Scanlon,* 473 U.S. 234 (1985).

In 1988 Congress passed the Fair Housing Amendments Act (42 U.S.C. 3601–3619), which prohibits discrimination against families with children and persons with disabilities. The law, which has been referred to as the most significant housing discrimination measure since the 1968 Civil Rights Act, was enacted in the midst of a presidential election when both candidates were eager to show their support for families and disabled people.

More important to future disability rights legislation, however, was that civil rights legislation had brought together groups that had fought discrimination on the basis of color, gender, and ethnicity. Now these activists were exposed to the types of discrimination faced by persons with disabilities, which forged an unexpected platform for what was to come. The Rev. Jesse Jackson, president of the National Rainbow Coalition, would later testify in a joint congressional hearing in support of the ADA, as would Representative Ron Dellums of California, representing the Congressional Black Caucus. The policy window was beginning to open.

United We Stand

As discussed in Chapter 4, one of the keys to the eventual success of the ADA was the combined efforts of two organizations: the Disability Rights Education and Defense Fund (DREDF) and the Consortium of Citizens with Disabilities (CCD). These advocacy groups operated in concert—but not through any central office of funding because each group within the coalition funded its own activities independent of one another. Early on, leaders agreed that they would work on a "class" concept: Groups representing specific disabilities or issues agreed to work on all of the issues affecting all persons with disabilities. The strategy was to keep the members of the disability rights movement united, rejecting any proposed change in the legislation that would exclude a particular group, such as people with mental illness.[20]

Another important early decision was to form coalitions between adults with disabilities and parents of children with disabilities. The parents had become mobilized in support of the Education for All Handicapped Children Act (EHA) of 1975 (20 U.S.C. 1232, 1401, 1405–1420, 1453), which had guaranteed the right of every child with a disability to free, appropriate education in the most integrated setting appropriate to the child's needs, as explained in chapter 2. Many of the families who had been involved in lobbying for the 1975 statute had already learned important political skills. The partnership also signified the intention of activists to change a model that traditionally had excluded participants other than those most directly affected by disability to speak for them.

Unification of purpose did not come easily and was built on a change in the role of the organizations themselves. Initially, most of the larger groups, such as the Association for Retarded Citizens and the National Easter Seals Society, considered their primary responsibility to be that of service provider. They aided specific constituents, such as disabled veterans, and often operated through local or regional chapters. In many cases, the national office of the organizations was in New York or another major city. Gradually, the mission and the headquarters changed. Constituent advocacy became the groups' driving force and Washington, D.C., their political home. Almost all of the national organizations began to hire lobbyists to press their issues onto the political agenda, establishing a presence in the nation's capital.[21]

DREDF was represented by Patrisha Wright, who had worked in the deinstitutionalization movement of the 1970s before joining the legal battle for civil rights for disabled people. Wright worked with senators Tom Harkin and Edward Kennedy to write a new version of the ADA that some advocates felt was much weaker than what was needed. Wright served as the pragmatic voice of the movement, however, recognizing the difficulty of gaining support for a bill that was bound to attract opposition from powerful business lobbies over the cost of its implementation.

Inclusion of people with AIDS and those who are HIV-positive under the ADA brought forth another coalition in support of the bill. The National Commission on AIDS brought together organizations with different political agendas who recognized the importance of ending discrimination. The Commission included medical groups such as the American Academy of Child and Adolescent Psychiatry, the American Medical Association, and the American Public Health Association. Church groups representing every point on the religious spectrum, such as the American Baptist Churches, USA, and the Episcopal Church, as well as the Synagogue Council of America, signed on. Native American groups supporting inclusion of AIDS under the ADA included the Pasgua Yuga Tribe, the Central Navajo AIDS Coalition, and the Phoenix Indian Service. Other constituencies represented were women (Women's Legal Defense Fund, Women's Equity Action League), ethnic minorities (National Puerto Rican Coalition, Community Service Council of Greater Harlem, Latinas AIDS Research Project), government associations (National Association of Counties), unions (AFL-CIO), and a host of public interest groups such as the Gray Panthers, Americans for Democratic Action, and the American Civil Liberties Union.

The religious lobby was of particular importance because representatives of various denominations and faith groups made clear their support for people diagnosed with AIDS and HIV. In a letter signed by representatives of dozens of organizations, the members explained the reason for their interest in the ADA: "As members of faith groups, it is our responsibility to strengthen and heal one another within the human family. The unity of the family is broken where any are left out or are subject to unequal treatment or discrimination."[22] Citing 1 Corinthians 12:26, one letter noted, "If one member suffers, all suffer together. If one member is honored, all rejoice together."

One early, somewhat unexpected alliance was forged with right-to-life groups that sought protection for disabled newborns who they believed might be at risk. In the early 1980s several cases reached the courts in which physicians or parents were alleged to have withheld treatment or ordered only the minimal level of care. The National Association for Retarded Citizens, among others, joined with these groups for a brief time as a way of broadening its base of support even though their ideologies often were quite different. Many disability activists were prochoice, and many people within the right-to-life movement opposed any further extension of federal power over the states. Both movements supported an amendment to the Child Abuse and Neglect Act of 1984 that directed states to establish procedures for investigating cases in which authorities suspected that treatment had been denied on the basis of disability.[23] As Richard Scotch notes, however, "The association between right-to-life and disability rights groups appears to have been an ad hoc alliance."[24]

Friends in High Places

Some observers believe that although the advocacy coalitions formed the grassroots support for the ADA, the presence of visible, powerful political leadership within the Democratic and Republican parties guaranteed its success. What brought many of the partisan forces together in support of the proposed law was "a hidden army" of individuals who were disabled themselves or had a family member who was disabled. Often, the disability was not well known or was kept secret from the public. Presidential Counsel C. Boyden Gray and disability rights attorney Evan Kemp shepherded the statute through to the Senate using their contacts within the White House and the disability rights movement. Gray himself was not disabled, but he had felt the prejudice against Southerners while growing up and understood some of the frustration of his disabled colleagues. Kemp, who had long been a friend to the president, had been diagnosed at age twelve with Kugel-Welander syndrome, a form of muscular dystrophy. Kemp became the director of the Disability Rights Center in 1980 and was a Republican insider who served as a speechwriter for President George H. W. Bush on disability issues. In 1990 Bush named Kemp as head of the Equal Employment Opportunity Commission, gaining praise for his friend's crackdown on workplace discrimination.

Iowa Senator Tom Harkin, who delivered part of a speech in sign language so his deaf brother could understand, joined Connecticut Senator Lowell Weicker, who had supported the first version of the law. Weicker lost his reelection bid in 1988 but continued to fight behind the scenes on behalf of his son, who has Down syndrome. Edward Kennedy's son had lost a leg to cancer, and his sister is retarded; the Kennedy family had long been supporters of rights for mentally retarded people, and the family had supported the Special Olympics for disabled athletes. Kansas Senator Bob Dole, who had been injured in World War II in a rescue mission in Italy, came forward, as did Utah's Orrin Hatch, whose brother-in-law had polio. Arkansas Senator Dale Bumpers told his colleagues that his daughter was paralyzed and in a wheelchair for six months, which sensitized him to something he had never before experienced.

In the House, Representative Tony Coehlo, who has epilepsy, had been the bill's original sponsor. When Coehlo left Congress after allegations that he had been involved in a controversial investment scheme, the mantle of leadership was placed on the shoulders of Maryland's Steny Hoyer— who, unknown to the press, had married a woman with epilepsy.

No doubt members of Congress also realized that there would be a potential political cost if they chose not to support the bill. Arkansas Senator David Pryor commented later, "It is very difficult, as all of us know, to even be perceived as possibly questioning any type of legislation that would be of assistance to the blind, the handicapped, the disabled, the elderly, the physically and the mentally impaired."[25] In that sense, framing the measure as a civil rights bill that covered people who had been discriminated against in the past seemed to be an ideal strategy.

Joseph Shapiro believes the most important, if not surprising, member of the "hidden army" was President Bush himself. His daughter Robin died of epilepsy in 1953, at the age of three. One of his sons, Neil, has a learning disability; another son, Marvin, wears an ostomy bag as a result of colon surgery. Bush's uncle John Walker had contracted polio, which ended his career as a surgeon. Bush gained surprising support at the 1988 Republican National Convention when, during his acceptance speech, he became the first presidential candidate to mention disability directly. "I'm going to do whatever it takes to make sure the disabled are included in the mainstream," he said—a move that would later bring many undecided disabled voters into the candidate's camp. Political pollster Louis Genevie remarked that "a candidate ignores the issues of disabled people at his own peril."[26]

LEGISLATIVE PROCESS

The 1988 election generated promises by both presidential candidates— Vice President George Bush and Massachusetts Governor Michael Dukakis—that they endorsed broad civil rights protections for people with disabilities. After Bush won the election handily, disability rights activists decided that the policy window had opened sufficiently for them to work toward another incarnation of the ADA. On May 9, 1989, Democrat Tom Harkin of Iowa and Minnesota Republican senator David Durenberger introduced legislation in the Senate, with Representatives Coehlo and Hamilton Fish jointly introducing a companion measure in the House in the 101st Congress. Bipartisan support was considered essential to gaining congressional approval for the bill, even though it had the underlying support of a Republican president and a Republican attorney general.

The legislative process in the Senate was considerably less complex than it was in the House. The Senate held its initial hearings before the Committee on Labor and Human Resources' Subcommittee on the Handicapped (subsequently renamed the Senate Subcommittee on Disability Policy). The measure, S. 933, went through additional hearings on May 10, May 16, and June 22 before going to markup on August 2. On the floor, the Senate passed the bill September 7, 1989, by a 76–8 vote, sending the measure on to the House.

In the House, the bill's key sponsors were Democrats Steny Hoyer of Maryland, who would coordinate the House stewardship of the bill; Major Owens of New York; John Dingell of Michigan; Norman Mineta and Don Edwards of California; and Republicans Hamilton Fish, Jr., of New York, Steve Bartlett of Texas, and Augustus Hawkins of California. Once introduced, the measure, H.R. 2273, faced a much more difficult legislative maze because it was considered by an unprecedented four full committees. Most of the debate occurred in the House Committee on Education and Labor's Subcommittee on Select Education, which held a joint hearing with the House Subcommittee on Employment Opportunities on July 18, 1989. Unlike the Senate, which held all of its meetings in Washington, D.C., the Committee on Education and Labor held meetings in Boston, Houston, and Indianapolis as well.

The House Committee on Energy and Commerce referred the bill to two separate subcommittees: the Subcommittee on Telecommunication and Finance, which held a hearing on September 27, 1989, and the Subcommittee on Transportation and Hazardous Waste, which held a hearing September 28. The third House committee to debate the proposed ADA was the Committee on the Judiciary's Subcommittee on Civil and Constitutional Rights, which held three hearings: August 3, October 11, and October 12 (with the full committee). Lastly, the House Committee on Public Works and Transportation's Subcommittee on Surface Transportation held two meetings (September 20 and September 26). House markup sessions followed a similar pattern, with the four full committees holding hearings from October 12, 1989, through May 2, 1990. The House voted on the bill May 17 and 22, 1990, where it passed by a vote of 403–20 before going to a conference committee.

The congressional debate over the ADA was based on a series of issues. In the Senate, for instance, Utah senator Orrin Hatch offered an amendment on the floor seeking to have a refundable tax credit of up to $5,000 to help small businesses comply with the public accommodations requirement of the bill. In his testimony, Hatch argued that although he supported serving persons with disabilities, he was concerned about small companies, such as sole proprietorships, that faced compliance difficulties. "We have to recognize that Federal requirements cost money and some of these people cannot afford to come up with that money."[27] Hatch's proposed amendment was countered by Texas senator Lloyd Bentsen, chair of the Senate Finance Committee, who pointed out that any Senate action that included a tax provision would be killed by the House, which jealously guards its role over fiscal matters. Article I, Section 7 of the U.S. Constitution says that any bill that raises revenue must originate in the House. Hatch argued, however, that his proposal was not a tax amendment and therefore was still germane to Senate action.

Costs were one of the key issues under debate. Several members argued that any form of tax credit for businesses would cost the federal government too much; others, such as Oregon senator Bob Packwood, pointed out that Congress has only rarely given tax credits for costs it imposes, such as for compliance with Occupational Safety and Health Administration regulations or air quality rules on emissions. Opponents of the tax credit also cited estimates that 51 percent of the accommodations that would have to be made would bear nominal costs, and an additional 30 percent of accommodations would cost less than $30. The tax credit amendment was defeated by a vote of 48–44. After this vote, one of the bill's chief supporters, Tom Harkin, chided Hatch for characterizing the vote as being anti-small business, as well as for not offering his amendment in committee. "A vote in favor of the amendment offered by the senator from Utah was a vote to kill this bill. Make no mistake about it, it was a vote to kill this bill," Harkin said. "We know that if this had been attached to this bill and went to the House, this bill would have gone nowhere."[28]

Another issue raised in both houses was a fear that passage of the ADA would lead to a flurry of lawsuits, most brought against small business owners who could little afford to litigate against an unhappy customer. One conservative publication asserted that ADA stood for "Attorneys' Dreams Answered."[29] The *Wall Street Journal* warned in an editorial that the proposed law was "loopy legislation" that would "mostly benefit lawyers who will cash in on the litigation that will force judges to, in effect, write the real law." Questioning President Bush's support for the ADA, the newspaper asked rhetorically, "Tom Harkin is one thing, but why would this White House so willingly dump such direct costs and a litigation nightmare on small and often struggling companies?"[30]

The definition of who would be covered by the term "disabled" led to some of the most confusing portions of the hearings on the ADA—in part because some members of Congress were not clear themselves on what constituted a disability. One senator seemed convinced that individuals who used illegal drugs would be considered disabled and read a list that included alcohol withdrawal, delirium, and hallucinosis. The question of whether homosexuality and bisexuality were disabilities also took up a considerable portion of the debate, despite assurances by the bill's sponsors that they were not included. Even after the final vote, Senator Jesse Helms of North Carolina questioned whether pedophiles, schizophrenics, kleptomaniacs, and transvestites would be considered disabled.

During June and July 1990, members of the conference committee held three more hearings before settling on a final version, which was passed by the House on July 12 by a 377–28 vote and by the Senate the following day, 91–6. The legislation became Public Law 101-336 on July 26, when President Bush signed the bill. Senator Harkin remarked that passage of the ADA was "one of the proudest days of his life" and credited former senator Lowell Weicker for his unflagging commitment to improving the quality of life for persons with disabilities. Senator Kennedy said the Senate's action marked "a historic step in the long journey to complete the unfinished business of America [to] bring full civil rights and fair opportunity" to all citizens. "Our message to America today is that disabled people are not unable. . . . Now, with this legislation, they will have a fair chance to participate in the mainstream of American life."[31]

STEALTH CAMPAIGN

Avoiding the media and any attempt to try to explain the legislation to the press became a key element of the fight for passage of the ADA. This tactic runs counter to conventional political wisdom on how to push the policy window open because the press usually is an essential element of the policy debate. Media scholar Martin Linsky argues, "When policymakers want to disseminate ideas about public issues, they hold press conferences, distribute press releases, leak information, and give speeches designed to receive press coverage."[32] In the case of the ADA, the media-avoidance strategy, described as "a heresy," was based on the belief that the media would be of little use to the disability rights movement. Joseph Shapiro, himself a journalist, explains: "The reason is that journalists have been too slow to understand the new civil rights consciousness of disabled Americans."[33] The lead lobbyist on the ADA, Patrisha Wright, noted, "We would have been forced to spend half our time trying to teach reporters what's wrong with their stereotypes of people with disabilities."[34]

As a result, media coverage of the legislative battle for the ADA was extremely limited, and only a handful of articles were published nationally. This lack of attention was in clear contrast to the years of coverage prior to the passage of the 1964 Civil Rights Act, which had been graphically presented by media around the world. Images of lynchings, police dogs, and fire hoses became synonymous with the struggle for civil rights; few parallel images characterized the needs of disabled persons. One exception—frequently repeated—was the March 1990 demonstration by members of ADAPT in Washington, D.C., described in chapter 4. The pictures of disabled persons attempting to crawl up the west front of the U.S. Capitol building nagged at Americans' conscience as no other scene in the movement's history. Shapiro cautions, however, that one of the dangers of being a stealth movement is that "in order to get attention activists must play on the very misunderstandings they are trying to erase. . . . Events like the 'crawl up' only confuse [reporters'] grasp on the issue."[35]

OPPOSITION FORCES

Few attempts at broadening civil rights protections have made it through the legislative process without opposition of some kind. Although the

ADA was no exception, it also was different. Sara Watson, for example, argues that attempts to guarantee civil rights for disabled persons never suffered from the stigma of affirmative action that had attached itself to other minorities. Attempts to improve the life conditions of blacks and women had created a backlash in the 1970s and 1980s even though affirmative action was designed to reduce the same kind of discrimination in employment, housing, and access to public services that disabled persons faced. The perception that nondiscrimination practices were taking jobs away from nonprotected classes, especially white males, has not ended. Watson also believes, however, that the disability rights movement had not evolved to the point that disabled people were considered a threat to the nondisabled majority. "The concept of providing civil rights protection for people with disabilities had advanced far enough to make itself palatable but not so far that it had become unpopular or even objectionable," Watson says.[36]

Although the final votes on the ADA might be perceived as reflecting overwhelming support for the measure, they fail to indicate the powerful political forces that opposed the bill and proposed amendments that disability advocates believed would significantly reduce its impact on civil rights. Some of the opposition came directly from industry trade associations that had specific concerns about the law's implementation (and they would later challenge its provisions in court). Other objections, however, were more ideological in nature, especially those raised by the conservative right.[37]

The National Federation of Independent Business, which represents more than a half-million small business owners, argued that the ADA was flawed because it allowed for "excessive penalties" and included other provisions that would make compliance particularly difficult for small business owners. The organization supported a tax credit to pay for the costs of accommodating disabled persons, on the grounds that provision of access should be shared by the general public.[38]

Other business organizations also attempted to weaken the law's provisions on the basis of cost. James DiLuigi, representing the American

Hotel and Motel Association, questioned members of the House about provisions requiring businesses to modify buildings for greater accessibility, arguing that the costs would be excessive. Similar testimony was offered by Christopher Hoey of the International Mass Retail Association.[39] Other groups that raised concerns about the accessibility provisions were the National Association of Theater Owners, the American Institute of Architects, the Minnesota Newspaper Association, and the Associated Builders and Contractors.

Part of the opposition was reflected in concerns over transportation that were discussed by the House Subcommittee on Surface Transportation. These concerns included cost estimates and implementation difficulties related to over-the-road buses, rural transit, and the ADA's accessibility requirements for small bus companies. Representatives from the New York City Metropolitan Transit Authority raised questions about costs, as did several members of the American Public Transit Association. Commuter rail system compliance issues were the subject of testimony by representatives of the Chicago Transit Authority; tour operators were represented by the National Tour Association.[40] Because of the overlapping jurisdictions among congressional committees, many similar issues about the modification of railroad passenger cars and stations for accessibility also were heard by the House Subcommittee on Transportation and Hazardous Waste. Amtrak officials warned that there would be difficulty in making rail transportation accessible, and they indicated doubts about their ability to meet modification deadlines proposed under the act.

Whatever salience these comments had before the members of Congress, however, they probably did not have the emotional appeal of the dozens of disabled persons who also testified, lobbied on behalf of the bill, or sat in the galleries listening to the debate. Some were famous, others were not. Muriel Lee related the problems she had as the mother of a disabled student (her son, Christopher). I. King Jordan, president of Gallaudet University, spoke about the significance of the ADA for deaf individuals. Lisa Carl, a young woman with cerebral palsy, told senators about a local movie theater that would not let her attend because of her disability. A woman who had breast cancer told of losing her job and being unable to find another one because she now had a history of the disease. People who could not come to Washington sent in their "discrimination diaries" and letters to document the discrimination they faced.

In signing the measure on July 26, 1990, President Bush noted, "I know there have been concerns that the ADA may be vague or costly, or may lead endlessly to litigation. But I want to reassure you right now that my administration and the United States Congress have carefully crafted this Act. We've all been determined to ensure that it gives flexibility, particularly in terms of the timetable of implementation; and we've been committed to containing the costs that may be incurred." He ended the signing ceremony with a phrase that has become a part of the cultural history of disability policy: "Let the shameful wall of exclusion finally come tumbling down."[41]

CHAPTER 6

The ADA as Policy

One of the words used frequently by supporters of the Americans with Disabilities Act is "promise." Activist Justin W. Dart, Jr., wrote that the law is "a promise to be kept. What is that promise? Whatever the act says legally, the clearly communicated promise of the ADA is that all people with disabilities will be fully equal, fully productive, fully prosperous, and fully welcome participants in the mainstream."[1]

Dart's vision of what the ADA was, or might become, has now been tempered by more than a decade. This chapter does not intend to quantify the impact of the law on elements of that promise. Instead, it seeks to describe objectively the process by which the law is being implemented by various agencies, the implementation and rulemaking stages of policymaking, enforcement of the statute, and the litigation that has resulted over questions about what the "promise" was intended to mean.

By design, this chapter includes a brief explanation of the provisions of the law, with an emphasis on how the five major titles have been implemented and adjudicated. Because there have been hundreds of rulemakings, settlement agreements, and court cases related to the ADA, this chapter draws attention to some of the most significant issues rather than attempting to provide a comprehensive analysis of the entire statute. That task is already underway through the work of other scholars and activists.[2]

PROVISIONS OF THE LAW

In terms of legislative complexity, the ADA ranks relatively low on the scale. It consists of just five major sections, called titles. Title I deals with discrimination in employment and affects employers (public and private) with fifteen or more employees. The statute requires employers to provide qualified individuals with a disability an equal opportunity to benefit from the full range of employment-related opportunities available to others. This includes the entire range of work activities, including recruitment and hiring, compensation and benefits, promotions, and social activities associated with the workplace. Title I also restricts the kinds of questions that can be asked of a potential employee related to disability before a job offer is made. One of the key provisions of this section is that employers make reasonable accommodations for disabled employees, unless those accommodations result in undue hardship for the employer. Charges of discrimination must be filed with the Equal Employment Opportunity Commission (EEOC) within 180 days;[3] individuals also may file a lawsuit in federal court once they receive a right-to-sue letter from the EEOC.

Title II affects all activities of state and local governments, with Subtitle B applying to transportation provided by public entities. This title requires state and local governments, regardless of size or funding, to give persons with disabilities an equal opportunity to benefit from all of their programs, services, and activities. This includes public meetings, recreational services, transportation, health care, voting, and other programs. To ensure equal opportunity, state and local governments must follow specific architectural standards in the construction of new buildings or when altering or remodeling older ones. If a building or service cannot be provided in an accessible form, the activity must be relocated to another location. Government entities also must make available devices to allow persons with disabilities to communicate effectively, including meeting notices through the provision of modified formats. Exemptions are possible only if there is a demonstration that the modification would fundamentally alter the nature of the service, program, or activity being provided or that it would result in undue financial and administrative burdens. The U.S. Department of Justice (DOJ) issues the implementing regulations for this title. Complainants also may seek redress through private lawsuits in federal court.

Complaints dealing with the transportation provisions of Title II (city buses, subways, commuter rail systems) are made through the Federal Transit Administration. Transportation authorities may not discriminate in the provision of their services and must make good-faith efforts to provide accessible vehicles and services.

Title III, Public Accommodations and Services Operated by Private Entities, affects all privately operated public accommodations, commercial facilities, and private entities offering certain examinations and courses, as well as privately operated transportation. The entities covered under Title III must comply with basic nondiscrimination requirements that prohibit exclusion, segregation, and unequal treatment and, as under Title II, assure disabled persons that their facilities and programs are accessible. Covered under Title III are restaurants, retail stores, hotels, movie theaters, private schools, convention centers, doctors' offices, homeless shelters, transportation depots, zoos, funeral homes, sports stadiums, and transportation providers such as taxi companies.

Sole responsibility for litigation rests with DOJ, using the remedies and procedures set forth in Section 204(a) of the 1964 Civil Rights Act. Alleged violations are investigated by the Attorney General, whose office may seek enforcement through a civil action in U.S. District Court. Individuals may file private actions under this title as well.

Telecommunication relay services and closed captioning are covered in Title IV, which is enforced by the Federal Communications Commission (FCC). The ADA requires that common carriers (such as telephone companies) make relay services available and accessible twenty-four hours a day, seven days a week. All federally funded public service announcements also must be closed-captioned for hearing-impaired persons. Complaints that involve intrastate telecommunications are handled by the state involved. If the state does not take action within 180 days, the FCC can reassert its jurisdiction.

Title V's miscellaneous provisions include the relationship of the ADA to other statutes, a requirement for provision of technical assistance, the role of the Architectural and Transportation Compliance Board (Access Board), and coverage of provisions to Congress. Although there are no specific enforcement structures, most cases of alleged discrimination are handled through the agencies responsible for compliance under Titles I, II, and III.

IMPLEMENTATION AND RULEMAKING

The simplicity and vagueness of the ADA have been an advantage and a curse. On one hand, the lack of specificity in several sections of the law probably helped secure its passage in Congress. Members who regarded the statute as one that simply guaranteed physical accessibility to facilities for persons in wheelchairs probably had no idea how the law might be interpreted. Even those who supported the measure appeared to be unaware of its implications and unintended consequences. Most of the opposition (described in chapter 5) came from parties who were concerned about the cost of the act's implementation. No one really understood the ultimate objective of the law—the elimination of discrimination.

As is often the case with pioneering legislation, the ADA's history has been shaped in large part by its implementation.[4] Jane West, a consultant who has served in various capacities as an advisor on disability policy, notes that passage of the law itself did not eliminate discrimination against persons with disabilities. Its implementation, she argues, was caught up in the politics of health care reform that dominated the first two years of the Clinton administration. In 1994, the president himself said that health care reform "would finish the business of the ADA. A more cynical observer commented, 'The administration won't aggressively enforce the ADA in the midst of courting the business community for support on health care reform.'"[5]

West says that the ADA's implementation also was enmeshed in the politics of unfunded mandates on business and on state and local governments. Although there was bipartisan support for the statute in Congress, concern over the law's regulatory timetable and, more important, its costs, were regarded as obstacles to be overcome. Without funding, implementation did not move forward at the pace many disability rights advocates had expected.

Researcher Andrew Batavia believes that the law's inability to substantially increase the numbers of persons with disabilities who are employed, educated, and socially active was predictable. "The policy assumptions of other components of our nation's disability policy, such as Social Security Disability Insurance and Supplemental Security Income programs, are still not consistent with those underlying the ADA. Moreover, the ADA was not designed to resolve all the problems experienced by people with disabilities."[6]

The implementation process has been directed by several agencies, depending on the specific title of the statute. As Box 1.1 shows, a myriad of federal departments and bureaus have been given some level of responsibility for the ADA.

Equal Employment Opportunity Commission

Section 106 of the ADA requires that the EEOC serve as the issuing agency for regulations implementing the Title I employment provisions of the law. The agency was the first to issue an Advance Notice of Proposed Rulemaking (ANPRM), on August 1, 1990—just a few days after President Bush had signed the law. It held only a short, one-month public comment period, receiving 138 comments, although 62 input meetings also were held at EEOC field offices. On February 28, 1991, the EEOC published a Notice of Proposed Rulemaking (NPRM) in the *Federal Register*, again with a one-month public comment period. This time, 697 comments were received and reviewed by the Commission staff, who noted that "the divergent views expressed in the public comments demonstrate the complexity of employment-related issues."[7]

The regulations were modeled on Section 504 of the Rehabilitation Act of 1973. One major change was to provide definitions for terms not previously defined in the regulations, such as "substantially limits," "essential functions," and "reasonable accommodation." Also added was interpretive guidance for persons with disabilities so that they could understand their rights, as well as to encourage compliance by covered entities. The final rule was published July 26, 1991—exactly one year after the signing of the ADA—and its regulations were made effective July 26, 1992.

U.S. Department of Justice

Like the EEOC, the Department of Justice published its final rule in the *Federal Register* on July 26, 1991, to implement provisions of Titles II and III.[8] The rule represented a year's worth of extensive negotiations and hearings to find ways of interpreting congressional intent on how state and local governments would comply with the new law. The short time frame was not especially burdensome because most programs and activities of state and local governments already had been covered by Section 504 of the Rehabilitation Act of 1973 and its amendments. Essentially, the new rules simply extended prohibitions against discrimination to governments that had not previously received federal financial assistance.

The implementation process is best understood by reviewing the rule-making history of the various titles of the ADA. DOJ published its NPRM on February 22, 1991, for Title III, and six days later published the NPRM for Title II. By the April 29, 1991, close of the public comment period for Title II, DOJ had received 2,718 comments. Four public hearings were held in spring 1991, at which 329 persons testified and 1,567 pages of testimony were compiled. The comments that DOJ received occupy almost six feet of shelf space and contain more than 10,000 pages; most were from individuals and organizations representing the interests of persons with disabilities. After these comments were analyzed by DOJ officials, the final rule was reviewed by the Office of Management and Budget (OMB).[9] The lengthier public comment period reflects the number of comments received and the potential impact of the regulations.

U.S. Architectural and Transportation Barriers Compliance Board

Among the most anticipated provisions of the ADA were requirements that facilities (public and private) be accessible to persons with disabilities. Advocates expected that the statute would serve as an impetus for facility managers and building owners to make the kinds of structural changes that had been discussed and recommended for the previous thirty years. The process of developing regulations to implement the accessibility provisions of the ADA was different in many ways, however, from those used by the EEOC and DOJ.

The issue of physical accessibility originally stemmed from a 1961 report from the President's Committee on the Employment of the Handicapped and the National Easter Seals Society for Crippled Children. The two groups published a nongovernmental guideline, "Specifications for Making Buildings and Facilities Accessible to and Usable by the Physically Handicapped." Their recommendations were adopted by the American National Standards Institute (ANSI) in October 1961 and served as the basis for subsequent statutory language.[10] Other accessibility guidelines were developed by nongovernmental groups such as the Building Officials and Code Administrators. Their involvement reflects the importance of professional individuals and organizations involved in the development of later standards and rules.

In 1961 the President's Committee was an advisory rather than a regulatory body, and its structure included an Architectural Barriers Committee that evaluated recommendations for removing architectural and environmental barriers. The Committee worked with ANSI and the Easter Seals Society to develop publications and to coordinate volunteer efforts around the country.

In 1965 Congress enacted amendments to the Vocational Rehabilitation Act that included a provision that authorized the creation of the National Commission on Architectural Barriers to Rehabilitation of the Handicapped, charged with preparing an overview and proposals to increase accessibility. By then, twenty-four states had taken some kind of official action to eliminate architectural barriers in public buildings. Disabled access was not generally considered when new buildings were being constructed, however, and there was limited community involvement in the decision-making process. No federal government-wide order had been issued to ensure elimination of barriers in the design and construction of federally assisted projects.[11]

A foreshadowing of just how difficult it would be to implement accessibility guidelines came after passage of the Architectural Barriers Act (ABA) of 1968, which gave power for standard setting to the General Services Administration (GSA) and the secretaries of Housing and Urban Development; Defense; and Health, Education and Welfare (now Health and Human Services). What made this phase of rulemaking somewhat unusual was that the GSA issued final rules without going through the traditional process of a public comment period.[12] The General Accounting Office (GAO) would later note, however, that the ineffectiveness of the ABA, and what it termed its "minor effect on making public buildings barrier free," was a result of "several language deficiencies which have lessened their effectiveness." The federal agencies that had been delegated authority to carry out congressional intent could easily circumvent the law by using their own interpretation of accessibility standards, could waive the standards on a case-by-case basis, and had complete discretion with regard to the nature or number of compliance surveys. Even the definition of the term "building," the GAO said, was deficient because it excluded many facilities from compliance.[13]

The U.S. Architectural and Transportation Barriers Board (Access Board) was created as a provision of the 1973 Rehabilitation Act. The Access Board was given a broad mandate by Congress—including ensuring that federal agencies complied with the ABA and its amendments, as well as studying ways of eliminating physical barriers and promoting use of the international accessibility symbol. The Access Board was given additional authority in 1978 when Congress enacted revisions to the Rehabilitation Act, and it became more representative of the disability community when President Jimmy Carter reconstituted its membership to include disabled persons. The election of Ronald Reagan as president brought a significant change in direction; in 1982, the Office of Management and Budget (OMB) recommended that the Access Board be eliminated, and other administration officials argued that the board was embarking on rules that imposed excessive regulatory compliance costs. From 1982 until the passage of the ADA in 1990, the Access Board grappled primarily with proposed minimum guidelines for accessibility—and little else.

Since then, the Access Board has focused on filling the gaps that developed as the full scope of the ADA has been explored. In 1991 the Access Board issued its first set of ADA Accessibility Guidelines (ADAAGs) for public and private buildings. As the guidelines began to be field tested, it became clear that revisions would become necessary. The Access Board's twenty-two-member ADAAG Review Advisory Committee—composed of representatives of the building industry, professional associations, state and local government officials, designers, architects, and disability advocates—began meeting in 1994 to update the guidelines and harmonize codes and standards throughout the United States.

Two issues illustrate the difficulties of implementing a law whose implications are still being uncovered: accessibility to outdoor recreation areas and standards for access to information technology. Unlike an amendment to the ADA itself, rulemaking by the Access Board involves changes to the ADAAGs rather than legislative action by Congress.

Although much of the attention surrounding the development of the law originally dealt with the built environment and accessibility to physical structures, it eventually became apparent that the law would have to deal with open spaces as well. What makes this issue especially interesting is that it grew out of the "reinventing government" movement adopted under the Clinton administration as part of the National Performance Review. The principle of regulatory negotiation, or "reg neg," for rulemaking[14] was designed as part of a package that would eliminate obsolete regulations; reward results, not red tape; get the decision-making process out of Washington; create grassroots partnerships; and negotiate, not dictate.[15]

Development of rules to deal with outdoor developed areas began with a set of recommendations from the Access Board published in July 1994 and was followed in June 1997 with the creation of a regulatory negotiation committee. The charge of the committee was to develop consensus accessibility guidelines for trails, picnic areas, camping facilities, and beaches.[16] The Access Board suggested the reg-neg process because there is a substantial amount of information about making recreation facilities accessible and remaining issues where there is no consensus are not well defined. One Access Board official told the committee's members that "the most critical issue for outdoor developed areas is balancing accessibility with the preservation of the fundamental nature of the outdoor recreation environments."[17] The committee was told from the outset that the scope of its work focused on design issues rather than program or policy issues, such as use of motorized vehicles within wilderness areas, use of interpreters in programs, and reservation policies on accessible camping sites. This limitation made the committee's duties more straightforward, and its members proceeded to fulfill their obligations as advisors.

For this type of rulemaking, the Access Board used a facilitator from the Federal Mediation and Conciliation Service. Meetings were held at various locations around the country; the process included site visits to beach access areas in Santa Cruz, California, as well as scheduled public comment periods. Much of the discussion was directed to technical specifications that would later be added to ADAAGs, such as the width of accessible routes to beaches and the rest-area interval for recreational trails. For this new rule, committee members relied not only on their own expertise but also on the experience of the U.S. Forest Service in making its trails accessible. Committee members then prioritized the areas they would address, beginning with picnic and camping facilities, followed by accessibility guidelines for trails. Gradually, the discussion expanded to define what constituted a picnic area, with committee members identifying more than thirty design elements. This list included not only picnic tables but water fountains, wheelchair storage spaces, interpretative displays, and public pay telephones.

Although the reg-neg process was designed to speed the process of consensus building, with the outcome representative of the respective constituent groups, rulemaking by any method is almost always a difficult and time-consuming process. The committee met ten times between June 1997 and July 1999, and work groups convened to gather information and develop recommendations for the full committee. The committee made its recommendations to the Access Board on September 15, 1999; a public comment period followed. Rather than making a decision at that point, the Access Board began to work on a cost-benefit analysis, which then had to be cleared by OMB. Further slowing implementation was a decision to hold an information meeting in conjunction with the National Recreation and Parks Association Congress in October 2001. Although this step did provide another opportunity for public comment, the proposed set of guidelines still had not been published by September 2002. The process, which began in July 1994, would take more than eight years to complete.

The Access Board acted much more quickly to implement guidelines related to the various means of disseminating information through electronic and information technology. Unlike the outdoor reg-neg committee's work, these rules were highly technical and opened up the need for standards that rarely had been considered prior to passage of the ADA. For many people with disabilities, the Internet and computers have opened up the world, allowing for access and integration that previously isolated millions of Americans (a topic discussed in greater depth in chapter 8). Under Section 508 of the 1973 Rehabilitation Act, the government is required to make all electronic and information technology in the federal sector accessible to persons with disabilities. The law applies to federal agencies when they develop, procure, maintain, or use such technology, and it was up to the Access Board to develop standards for procurement and accessibility. The standards also were folded into the regulations for federal procurement policies that govern the Federal Acquisition Regulatory Council. The standards define the types of technology covered and lay out the minimum level of access required, along with compatibility with adaptive equipment that people with disabilities commonly use for information and communication access. This includes a wide range of products, including Braille displays, screen readers, software applications and operating systems, web-based information or applications, telecommunication products, video and multimedia products, self-contained closed products (information kiosks, copiers, printers, calculators, facsimile machines), and desktop and portable computers. Compliance is required except where the regulations would pose an "undue hardship"; technologies related to national security are exempt, as are products procured before June 21, 2001.

One of the reasons that web accessibility rose to the top of the policy agenda is that technology has advanced rapidly to provide information without an internationally accepted standard for minimal web accessibility. Executive Director of the International Center for Disability Resources on the Internet Cynthia Waddell notes that unless a website is designed in an accessible format, "significant populations will be locked out as the World Wide Web rapidly advances from a text-based communication format to a robust, graphical format embracing audio and video clip tools."[18] DOJ's Office of Civil Rights has further defined what constitutes "effective communication" through the Internet as "timeliness of delivery, accuracy of the translation, and provision in a manner and medium appropriate to the significance of the message and the abilities of the individual with the disability."[19]

To implement the law, the Access Board created the Electronic and Information Technology Access Advisory Committee, composed of twenty-seven representatives from industry, disability organizations, and other interested parties. Initial standards were proposed on March 31, 2000, with a sixty-day public comment period that resulted in more than 100 submissions. The final standards were issued on December 21, 2000, becoming effective June 21, 2001—just more than a year after they were proposed. The regulations include an administrative process that allows persons with disabilities to file complaints concerning the accessibility of an agency's electronic or information technology or the alternative route of filing a civil action against an agency.[20] Even before the guidelines were accepted, the Access Board began to develop technical assistance and training materials on the new standards. A private firm was awarded a contract to develop fact sheets, brochures, guides on how to make websites accessible to people with disabilities, and training modules for various audiences.[21] Bobby—a website that will perform a free accessibility diagnostic and make suggestions— is one of many that helps webmasters make their sites accessible.

No doubt the Access Board, like other organizations, has developed its own learning curve as it deals with issues perhaps never envisioned by the ADA's sponsors. The hearings on the ADA never covered questions such as how to make amusement rides, golf courses, swimming pools, or boating facilities fully accessible. Nor was there extensive discussion on how to provide access to swing sets and teeter-totters or soft, contained play structures made of plastic, netting, and fabric. Since passage of the ADA, the Access Board has dealt with dozens of similar unforeseen topics, including construction and alteration of detention and correctional facilities, children's play areas and equipment, over-the-road buses, water passenger vessels, sports and recreation facilities, accessible sidewalks, traffic signals and intersections, and public rights-of-way.

The Access Board also is in the process of revising the ADAAGs on the basis of more than 2,500 comments, most of them from persons with disabilities.[22] At a public forum celebrating the ten-year anniversary of the ADA, the Access Board heard requests from the audience to deal with multiple chemical sensitivities, the relationship between the board's guidelines and building codes and standards, and access to polling places, movie captioning, and visual alarms.[23] Forums, websites, and public hearings continue to uncover additional needs that were not addressed by the legislation and have been left open to interpretation and, ultimately, more rulemaking. Because the ADAAG is so critical to implementation of the law itself, its revision probably would be a much more lengthy process than the development of specific regulations.

Not all of the Access Board's actions have been codified in rules. In 1999 the Access Board joined with the American National Standards Institute (ANSI) and the Acoustical Society of America to develop a new standard for classroom acoustics. The partnership was based on studies that show that high levels of background noise adversely affect learning environments. This issue is of particular concern for young children who require optimal conditions for reading and comprehension. Although the standards are voluntary through ANSI, they may become part of state and local building codes.[24]

The Access Board began to investigate complaints related to the ABA in 1976. In its first twenty-five years, more than 3,300 complaints were investigated, about one-third of which involved post offices (of which there are more than 38,000 in the United States). When the Access Board works with other agencies to investigate complaints, it relies on the 1984 Uniform Federal Accessibility Standards, which are similar to the ADAAGs. The goal is to make the two sets of standards congruent so that there is uniform access, especially when a facility is subject to both the ABA and the ADA.[25]

Other Agencies and Commissions

Implementation also has been facilitated through various state agencies and commissions, which have worked on a more informal basis to make sure that the rights of disabled persons are protected under the ADA. Cases often have been dealt with on a state or local basis without going through the formal complaint process. For instance, in 1992 a disabled veteran and activist, Robert Reuter, filed a complaint with the Maryland Commission on Human Relations because he was unable to get his wheelchair aboard the 1854 warship Constellation. The vessel is the last all-sail warship built for the U.S. Navy and is being restored at a cost of more than $9 million by the Constellation Foundation. In settling the complaint, the foundation agreed to provide a hand-cranked portable lift between the ship's top deck and gun deck, along with videotaped tours and other alternative visual experiences for areas that cannot be made physically accessible. Initial estimates placed the expected costs at $100,000 for the renovations and modifications, which require no electricity and no permanent attachment to the ship.

A spokesperson for the Maryland commission expressed his pleasure at the agreement, which did not require court action or additional costs for the complainant. "It advances the rights of persons with disabilities—their rights of access to historic properties—while at the same time respecting the need to protect historically significant properties from damage, destruction, or alterations."[26]

ENFORCEMENT

Political scientists Donald Van Meter and Carl Horn, two of the pioneers in the study of implementation, identify two types of enforcement follow-up activities that are most important in the context of interorganizational or intergovernmental relations. First, technical advice and assistance can be provided. Van Meter and Horn note that higher-level officials often can do a great deal to facilitate implementation by aiding subordinates in interpreting federal regulations and guidelines, structuring responses to policy initiatives, and obtaining physical and technical resources required to carry out a policy. Second, federal officials can rely on positive and negative sanctions to gain compliance. This may involve anything from providing grant funds to other parties to gentle and explicit forms of coercive power.[27]

Six years after the ADA was signed, civil rights attorney Timothy M. Cook reminded his fellow advocates that if the act were administered and enforced in a manner similar to previous disability rights statutes, the legacy of discrimination and segregation would not be dealt with "root and branch as Congress intended." Cook predicted that if federal agencies charged with implementing the law did not take the necessary actions to carry out the directives of the ADA, the law would be allowed "to accompany its legislative predecessors languishing in the hollows of non-enforcement."[28]

Since 1990 several public and private agencies, scholars, and advocacy groups have attempted to evaluate the law's impact on the basis of the number of enforcement actions and subsequent litigation. One of the most comprehensive evaluations was conducted by the National Council on Disability (NCD), the independent federal agency that has a congressional mandate for monitoring implementation and compliance. As part of the ten-year anniversary of the signing of the law, the NCD issued three separate reports under its series "Unequal Protection Under Law." The first report, released in March 1999, was *Enforcing the Civil Rights of Air Travelers with Disabilities: Recommendations for the Department of Transportation and Congress;*[29] the second was *Back to School on Civil Rights.*[30] These reports were followed in June 2000 by *Promises to Keep: A Decade of Federal Enforcement of the Americans with Disabilities Act.*[31] The NCD reports credit the ADA with transforming the social fabric of the nation and bringing the principle of disability civil rights into the mainstream of public policy. They also note that the ADA has become an international symbol of the promise of human and civil rights and a blueprint for policy development in other countries. Yet all three reports characterize implementation with phrases such as "lack of leadership" and "insufficient resources," placing primary blame on the federal agencies charged with enforcement and policy development.

The NCD's June 2000 report said the agencies have been, to varying degrees, "overly cautious, reactive, and lacking any coherent and unifying national strategy. Enforcement efforts are largely shaped by a case-by-case approach based on individual complaints rather than an approach based on compliance monitoring and a cohesive, proactive enforcement strategy." The report goes on to note that the leadership and enforcement deficiencies appear to be related to the "culture" of particular bureaucracies that have hewed to their traditional mission and circumspectly defined their constituency, undermining federal enforcement of the ADA. "Their net impact has been to allow the destructive effects of discrimination to continue without sufficient challenge in some quarters. Arguably, the major impact of this weak enforcement environment has been its contribution to the problematic federal court interpretations of key ADA principles that have unjustly narrowed the scope of the law's protections."[32]

One of the criticisms leveled in the report was against the Department of Transportation, which has six quasi-independent units responsible for enforcing the transportation provisions of the ADA. The NCD notes inconsistencies in the way the statute is interpreted, the approach to complaint investigation, and the priority placed on public education, with some units having broad discretion in meeting the law's accessibility requirements and timetables. The report also criticizes the agencies' response to inaccurate and misleading negative media portrayals of the statute, which are said to have "undermined public support for ADA, caused a backlash against the expansion of the civil rights of individuals with disabilities, and perhaps fostered a perception that noncompliance was not an unreasonable response to an 'excessive' mandate. The absence of strong and visible federal government leadership has contributed to the concern that there is little balance in the public discourse on ADA and a general public misunderstanding of the aims and requirements of ADA."[33]

The report's general conclusion cites the lack of coordination: "Had all the federal agencies worked more closely in collaboration with each other and stakeholders on developing a national strategy, ADA would be in a much stronger position as we mark the tenth anniversary of its passage. . . . The overall record indicates that the enforcement agencies have been hesitant to exercise leadership in litigating difficult or controversial issues, or to maintain sufficiently rigorous positions in settlement negotiations."

LITIGATION

Another way of looking at the ADA's implementation is by analyzing court cases, most of which are filed by plaintiffs in federal district courts. In one study of Title I (employment), researcher Ruth Colker found that from June 1992 to July 1998, courts of appeals had issued decisions in 475 cases. By comparison, only 25 Title III cases had reached the appellate courts during that same period.[34]

Studies of court decisions alone are misleading because DOJ participates in several other enforcement procedures. Settlement agreements probably are the most common method, but it is difficult to determine exactly how many agreements are reached because many remain confidential. DOJ does publish the general results of its actions on a public website, but there are no reliable statistics on any of its remedies. Unlike many types of litigation, the ADA is commonly enforced and violations are remedied when a losing party agrees to end discriminatory practices, without a claim for financial compensation. These complaints involve forms of injunctive relief, where the costs of settling are borne by the federal government without the necessity of a trial.

Typical is a case brought to DOJ in 1994, in which complainants, who are deaf, filed under Title II of the ADA against the Oakland, California, police department. The complaint alleged that police department staff failed to provide them with access to a telecommunications device for the deaf (TDD) and that they were needlessly incarcerated because they could not communicate with persons who might assist them. The parties reached a four-page settlement agreement in 1998 that spelled out very specifically the actions that the police department agreed to take voluntarily, including development of a written policy on provision of interpreting services, distribution of the new policy to all police officers, and training on how to operate TDDs.[35]

One of the myths that surround the statute is that plaintiffs will bring a cause of action as a way of "making big bucks" in a high-profile complaint. Some cases that go to trial do involve financial reward—usually when an individual with a disability has suffered some form of physical injury. According to one study, when a plaintiff suffered a serious injury as a result of faulty accessibility standards and sued for damages under the cause of negligence, the typical award was about $10,000, although one individual was awarded $512,000. That case involved a suit against a physician and a hospital for the failure to admit the plaintiff to the hospital in violation of the ADA.[36]

Much more difficult to resolve are cases involving "stigmatic harm"—situations in which there is no physical harm to the plaintiff. In these situations, an individual may suffer embarrassment, emotional distress, humiliation, or other nonphysical harm; as many cases suggest, however, it is difficult for a judge or jury to determine what level of compensation is appropriate. Unlike cases of racial discrimination, in which courts have had less reluctance to order awards when an individual was refused service or access to a facility,[37] there is still a sense that the kind of emotional damage suffered by a person with a disability is less severe.

How does one determine the level of emotional harm to a disabled person? In a 1998 settlement agreement against the Holiday Inn and Crowne Plaza hotel chains, complainants argued that the accessible rooms they had reserved in advance were not available when they arrived at the hotel, which one DOJ official said "can be a disaster for a family vacation." In a mediated settlement, the owner of the hotel chains agreed to set up a mediation program to resolve complaints about access, conduct an inventory of accessible rooms and equipment, train hotel employees, and keep an ADA-trained architect on staff to assist with renovations. The forty-eight people who filed complaints shared a $75,000 financial award—little recompense in comparison to awards for other types of complaints.[38]

Putting a price on the lack of access often is not considered when the level of harm is being determined. An example is a settlement agreement reached in 1998 involving approximately 3,000 Shell gas stations. The class-action complaint against the company resulted in an agreement that requires gas stations across the country to conduct accessibility surveys and make significant accessibility improvements to all areas of the stations where needed. The company also agreed to provide training and implement policies that will be of assistance to their customers with disabilities. There is no way, however, of quantifying how much disabled customers suffered because they could not use the station's pumps and other facilities.[39]

It is important to note that it is only under Title III that the DOJ has statutory authority to seek civil damages if it brings suit, and the level of compensation is set by law. Colker found that only forty-six settlements had been reached in Title II cases as of September 1998, which represents approximately six years of enforcement. DOJ obtained a significant civil fine of $50,000 in only one case; in the other sixteen in which monetary settlements had been reached, the amounts ranged from $250 to $10,000. Two of the fines were in the form of gift certificates of $500 and $900.[40] Clearly, settlement agreements provide little financial incentive for persons filing complaints under Title III.

What activists find even more disturbing is that it appears that some defendants who are sued under Title III would rather fight than comply.

In Whitefish, Montana, the management of the Ptarmigan Village resort spent more than $50,000 in a battle against a couple who live in one of the resort's condominiums. Both use wheelchairs, and they opposed a proposal by the management of the condo association to put wood chips on the paths throughout the common areas. A meeting was held, but in an inaccessible location—"deliberately and maliciously," the couple's attorney said. A second meeting was scheduled in full view of the resort's staff and guests, making the couple feel intimidated and exposed.

Once the lawsuit was filed, the couple was required by the resort's attorneys to provide written answers to a series of questions about their disability, including "the number of inches above the knee of your amputation for your right and left leg," along with detailed descriptions of every set of prosthetics worn. The association board's president said in a deposition that if it were not for the lawsuit, "we would be working, I believe, cooperatively . . . to make accommodations and resolve problems." One observer believes that the resort's owners believe they can ignore or dismiss the couple's concerns because they argue that they are not subject to the provisions of the ADA. "They seem intent on shaping a case for a Montana jury that likely knows little to nothing about disability rights by painting [the couple] as complainers who simply are not trying hard enough physically, but demanding special concessions they do not deserve."[41]

In the years since the ADA was signed into law, there have been hundreds of court cases filed against defendants who have failed to properly implement the statute. Despite the federal government's attempts to keep enforcement out of the judicial arena, it has now become clear that litigation is becoming a primary tool of the disability rights movement and, to many advocates, the only way to assure that the civil rights of disabled people will be protected. Much of that litigation has come with the formation of public interest law firms dedicated to expanding the civil rights of persons with disabilities and their families.

One of the most prominent national law centers is the Disability Rights Education and Defense Fund (DREDF), which grew out of the Berkeley independent living center in the mid-1970s. Originally called the Disabled Paralegal Advocacy Program, it began with a staff of volunteers; eventually these volunteers were replaced by attorneys, and the organization became the Disability Law Resource Center, incorporating in 1979 as DREDF. It used as its model similar civil rights groups such as the NAACP Legal Defense and Education Fund.

The organization was prominent in several of the key legal victories of the 1980s, representing disabled plaintiffs and acting as a resource for others. Attempts by the Reagan administration to weaken the regulations adopted under Section 504 of the Rehabilitation Act of 1973 and the 1975 Education for All Handicapped Children Act were opposed by DREDF staff members who provided training and workshops for disability advocates. DREDF also helped to draft the ADA and worked actively to lobby in support of the legislation. The organization established a Clinical Legal Education Program, and it operates a *pro bono* panel and a lawyer referral service and provides technical assistance through funding by DOJ.[42] Other public interest law firms include the Disability Rights Center (founded and funded initially by Ralph Nader's Center for the Study of Responsive Law to protect the rights of consumers of durable medical equipment) and the Legal Action Center, which focuses on protecting persons with histories of alcoholism, drug dependence, and AIDS.

Much of the reason for the use of litigation as a strategy has been the success rate of public interest law firms that have taken on controversies of "David and Goliath" proportions. In 1993 the nonprofit group Disability Rights Advocates (DRA) was founded in Oakland, California, as a way of ensuring enforcement of the ADA. Laurence W. Paradis, a cofounder of the law center, notes that although the ADA was indeed landmark legislation for people with disabilities, "the reality is that discrimination against us remains pervasive and cannot be overcome by legislation alone."[43] Other major cases have been brought by state-level protection and advocacy (P&A) firms.

Resorting to litigation, however, challenges traditional theories about whether a disabled litigant has a good chance of winning a case in the courtroom. In 1974 Marc Galanter's pioneering study of litigation and social change delineated the theory of party capability, in which he argued that the "haves" (who tend to be repeat players in the courts) tend to come out ahead of the "have nots" in litigation. Litigants with the greatest resources and the lowest relative stakes have the highest rate of success, Galanter argued, particularly when they are matched against individual litigants.[44] Other studies have sought to identify why the "haves" are more likely to prevail and have found that a variety of factors are responsible, from the advantage of hiring better lawyers to experience and wealth. One study of U.S. Courts of Appeals found that the overall success rates of governments were about four times as high as the success rates of individuals and one and a half times the success rates of businesses.[45]

A recent study of individual litigants with relatively low levels of resources found, however, that the disparity in success rates can be reduced by the intervention of interest groups that will support their position with the filing of an *amicus curiae* brief. The researchers found that this is especially true of "have nots" (such as persons with disabilities); these litigants tended to be more successful because they benefited from the combined expertise and experience of attorneys who previously had represented clients in similar circumstances.[46] Such findings represent one of the major trends in litigation in disability-related cases—the pooling of resources.

A second trend in ADA litigation is characterized by the deliberate choice of defendants. Rather than filing suit against an individual store owner for failure to implement Title III of the law, for instance, public interest law firms have chosen companies and organizations with deep pockets whose losses in court will serve as a financial and public relations burden. DRA, for example, filed a class-action suit against the San Francisco Housing Authority for its failure to provide accessible housing. The case began with a teenage plaintiff living with his family who had repeatedly requested basic access features, including a ramp into his apartment. Paradis notes that by filing suit against the Housing Authority as a class action, DRA was able to enforce immediate access for the plaintiff, as well as forcing the agency to modify hundreds of other units that, under federal law, should have been accessible years before.[47]

Subsequently, DRA (sometimes in conjunction with other firms) took on other major players, including the Oakland, California, school district, the city of San Francisco, San Francisco's MUNI bus system, Greyhound Bus Lines, Boston University, San Francisco State University, the United Parcel Service, the Bay Area Rapid Transit System, and the California State Department of Parks and Recreation and the State of California for failing to make its 263 parks and facilities accessible. Similar actions have been brought by public interest firms and advocates against the Greater Baltimore Medical Center, the Amoco chain of gas stations, and the Hard Rock Cafe.

Along with defendants with deep pockets, litigation has sometimes focused on "celebrity" cases involving well-known or highly publicized persons who have faced discrimination. By representing a high-profile complainant, law firms garner additional attention and media coverage.

Pauline Horvath was a civilian working at Alameda Naval Aviation Depot in California in 1982 when she started work as one of the first disabled employees ever hired by the Navy. Horvath, who has rheumatoid arthritis, was promoted six times in six years, and her boss readily installed new ramps to help her get around in her wheelchair, which she used for long-distance travel. In May 1988 a new boss walked into Horvath's office and said, "It's my office, and I don't want a wheelchair in it." Horvath moved her wheelchair to a closet down the hall and hobbled painfully on crutches. Her supervisor said she was concerned the wheelchair could block employee access; she also forbade Horvath to use a speaker phone, forcing Horvath to answer the telephone by knocking the receiver off the hook and placing her head on the desk so she could speak into it. A second-level supervisor also refused to accommodate Horvath, stating in writing that Horvath's wheelchair was similar to a golf cart.

In 1997, after the Navy refused to grant any of the accommodations Horvath requested to help her continue working, she sued the Navy, initially asking for $30,000 in compensatory damages. The story of the Navy's actions, which Horvath terms "outrageous," was passed along to disabled activists and, eventually, to the media. After the word was out, the Navy agreed to a $300,000 settlement, and the Navy allegedly offered even more if Horvath agreed to keep quiet about the case. None of the Navy officials involved in the case were ever disciplined, and a short time later the naval station closed down. The U.S. attorney representing the Navy said that "because the service admitted the discrimination in its own report, there was nothing the Navy could do but settle."[48]

KEY LITIGATION ISSUES

Prior to 1998, virtually all of the cases that were not settled out of court ended at the Circuit Court level, with the U.S. Supreme Court "deciding not to decide" ADA cases. Between 1998 and 2001, however, the Supreme Court chose to grant *certiorari* in an unprecedented number of cases, which some observers believe have only further complicated and confused American disability policy. These cases have made the statute more visible and reignited many of the debates over discrimination of disabled persons. As the sampling of issues and cases in Box 6.1 shows, there were only eight major cases heard by the Court in the eleven years after the ADA was enacted, and none before 1998.

Constitutionality and Applicability of the ADA

Prior to 2000, several claimants attempted to force the U.S. Supreme Court to rule on whether the ADA was constitutional. In *Pennsylvania Department of Corrections v. Yeskey,* 524 U.S. 206 (1998), state officials challenged whether Title II of the ADA is applicable to state prison systems, and the Supreme Court agreed that prisons were not exempt. Most filed cases that reached the U.S. Circuit Courts of Appeal dealt with whether Congress had the authority to waive individual states' sovereign immunity when the law was enacted. One of these cases, *Alsbrook v. City of Maumelle, Arkansas,* 184 F. 3d 999 (8th Cir. 1999), was granted *certiorari* and was scheduled for oral arguments on April 26, 2000, but was dismissed on March 2 of that year because the parties reached a settlement.

BOX 6.1

Major U.S. Supreme Court Cases Interpreting the Americans with Disabilities Act, 1990–2002

1998   *Pennsylvania Dept. of Corrections v. Yeskey,* 524 U.S. 206
            (June 15, 1998)
            Applicability of the ADA to individuals in state prisons
            Bragdon v. Abbott, 524 U.S. 624 (June 25, 1998)
            Discrimination against person with HIV seeking dental
            treatment

1999   *Cleveland v. Policy Managements Systems Corp.,* 526 U.S. 799
            (May 24, 1999)
            Applicability of ADA to person filing for SSDI
            Olmstead v. L.C., 527 U.S. 581 (June 22, 1999)
            Provision of services in the most integrated setting appropriate
            to the needs of qualified persons with disabilities
            Sutton v. United Airlines, Inc., 527 U.S. 471 (June 22, 1999)
            Applicability of ADA to persons with correctable vision
            condition
            Murphy v. United Parcel Service, 527 U.S. 516 (June 22, 1999)
            Applicability of ADA to person with high blood pressure
            Albertsons, Inc. v. Kirkinburg, 527 U.S. 555 (June 22, 1999)
            Definition of disabled for person with monocular vision

2001   *Board of Trustees of the University of Alabama v. Garrett,* 531 U.S.
            356 (February 21, 2001)
            Applicability of Title I to state government employees seeking
            monetary damages
            PGA Tour, Inc. v. Martin, 532 U.S. 661 (May 29, 2001)
            Applicability of Title III to qualified entrants in professional golf
            tournaments

2002   *Toyota Motor Mfg. v. Williams,* 122 S.Ct 681 (January 8, 2002)
            Narrows definition of disability to substantial limitation in
            performing manual tasks
            US Airways v. Barnett, No. 00-1250 (April 29, 2002)
            Seniority system and relationship to reasonable accommodation

Chevron v. Echazabal, No. 00-1406 (June 10, 2002)
Employer refusal to hire disabled person because of health threat
to employee
Atkins v. Virginia, No. 00-8452 (June 20, 2002)
Executions of mentally retarded criminals are "cruel and unusual
punishment" prohibited by Eighth Amendment to U.S.
Constitution

At almost the same time, the Supreme Court granted *certiorari* in *Garrett v. University of Alabama at Birmingham Board of Trustees,* 193 F.3d 1214 (11th Cir. 1999), a case similar to *Alsbrook.* Disability advocates were especially concerned about the direction the Court might take because it previously had held that Congress did not have authority to apply the Age Discrimination in Employment Act to the states.[49] The facts surrounding the case and the impact of the ruling in *Garrett* are discussed in detail in the Epilogue. It is one of the most important U.S. Supreme Court rulings since the ADA was enacted.

Reasonable Accommodation

The phrase "reasonable accommodation" usually is applied to work environments where a person with a disability is entitled to equal employment opportunities, requiring that employers must try to find a reasonable accommodation that would allow the person to perform the essential functions of the job. The difficulty faced by the courts has been the term "reasonable"; also at issue has been whether an employer attempts to comply in nonwork facilities such as cafeterias and restrooms, as well as job restructuring or physical accessibility.

Most cases related to reasonable accommodation have been heard by federal courts of appeal. In a 1996 case, the appellate court ruled that "reasonableness" depends on the individual circumstances of each case. The ruling underscored the commonly accepted principle that reasonable accommodation requires a fact-specific, individualized analysis of the disabled person's circumstances and the accommodations that might allow the person with a disability to meet the program's standards.[50] This analysis is the basis for the U.S. Supreme Court's ruling in *PGA, Inc. v. Casey Martin* (also discussed in the Epilogue).

Undue Hardship

Using language originally included in regulations promulgated by the federal Department of Health, Education and Welfare (now Health and Human Services), the ADA provides that under Title I an employer may claim exemption if the reasonable accommodation for a disabled employee becomes an undue hardship. When the language appeared in the 1973 Rehabilitation Act, it was considered an "inconspicuous" part of the legislation.[51]

As opposition to the ADA began to grow in the late 1980s, however, many of the critics seemed to be convinced that virtually any accommodation would constitute an undue hardship, especially to small businesses. Subsequent research has found that this is rarely true and that in fact there are economic benefits to employing persons with disabilities.[52] Two studies—one in 1994 and the other in 1996—found that in a sample of a company with more than 300,000 employees, the 600 workplace accommodations required little or no cost; the average direct cost was less than $30.[53] The U.S. Supreme Court had not ruled on this issue by the end of its 2001–2002 session.

Integration Mandate

The most prominent U.S. Supreme Court case dealing with this language in the ADA is *Olmstead v. L.C.*, 119 S.Ct. 617 (1999). Two women with mental disabilities charged that the state failed to provide them with treatment in the most integrated setting according to their needs. This highly publicized case, which is discussed in more detail in chapter 7, became the subject of nationwide rallies, candlelight vigils, and Internet protests. It resulted in a split, and confusing, decision that is likely to lead to more litigation on what Congress actually intended.

Defining Disability

The ADA defines a disability in terms of three factors: a physical or mental impairment that substantially limits one or more of the major life activities of an individual; a person with a record of such an impairment; or one who is regarded as having such an impairment.[54] Initially the concept of impairment was interpreted broadly, encompassing physiological disorders or conditions, cosmetic disfigurement, or anatomical loss, along with mental or psychological disorders. In one Nebraska case, a two-day migraine headache occurring every one or two months was considered an impairment because it was severe and debilitating.[55] In a circuit court ruling, a police department's decision to discharge a diabetic police officer was upheld because the individual failed to monitor his condition to allow him to function. The court interpreted the ADA as requiring persons seeking protection under the statute to attempt to control their disability.[56]

One of the initial Title III cases in the Supreme Court that helped define the rights of a person with a disability was *Bragdon v. Abbott,* 524 U.S. 624 (1998), in which a dentist refused, outside a hospital setting, to fill the cavity of a person who was HIV-positive. The dentist argued that he would be at undue risk of contracting a life-threatening illness if the patient were not treated in a hospital setting and that he had the right not to treat her at all because she was not defined as a person with a disability. The patient, however, argued that she was entitled to the ADA's protection even though she was asymptomatic because HIV interfered with the major life activity of reproduction. In this test case of Title III protections, the courts concluded that Abbott was an individual with a disability and therefore was entitled to injunctive relief.

Four cases decided more recently have focused attention on the definition of disability. In *Cleveland v. Policy Management Systems Corp.,* 119 U.S. 1597 (1999), the Supreme Court was asked to decide whether a person who has applied for Social Security Disability Insurance is presumed not to be a "qualified individual" under the ADA and therefore barred from suing for job discrimination. A unanimous Court ruled that application for, or receipt of, SSDI benefits does not automatically bar a claim of discrimination. In *Sutton v. United Airlines,* 119 S.Ct. 2139 (1999), the Court ruled against twin sisters with severe nearsightedness who applied to be pilots and claimed discrimination when they were not hired. The Supreme Court, in agreement with a lower court's ruling, found that they were not covered by the ADA because their vision is correctable.

Vaughn Murphy, a United Parcel Service mechanic, lost his case, in which he claimed a disability because of hypertension. As in the *Sutton* case, the Court found that the plaintiff was not disabled because his high blood pressure could be treated with proper medication.[57] Lastly, *Albertsons, Inc. v. Hallie Kirkinburg* (No. 98-0591) questioned whether a person with monocular vision is a person with a disability under ADA. Kirkinburg, a truck driver, sued the grocery store company after he was fired, claiming protection under the ADA. The Court ruled against Kirkinburg, further narrowing the definition of what constitutes a disability by denying him relief.

Several attorneys and civil rights advocates have expressed alarm at the Supreme Court's narrowing of the application of the ADA. Arlene Mayerson, directing attorney for DREDF, and Matthew Diller, associate professor of law at Fordham University, note that "For many people with disabilities, the recent rulings of the Supreme Court slam the door that Congress and President Bush opened."[58] The two claim that the Court's rulings on the definition of disability erect barriers to individuals whose disabilities are mitigated or controlled by technical aids or medical treatment. "When it comes to the ADA, the Court just doesn't 'get it.'"[59]

Physical and Programmatic Accessibility

For various reasons, covered entities have attempted to convince the courts that they should be exempt from portions of the ADA that require physical and programmatic accessibility. In *People of New York ex rel. Spitzer v. County of Delaware,* 82 F. Supp. 2d 12 (N.D.N.Y. 2000), the court ruled that a county that had failed to provide accessible polling places for citizens with disabilities was required to do so. A similar ruling, relating to the accessibility of a county courthouse, found that the county had violated the provisions of the ADA.[60] Although most cases have focused on physical accessibility, in New Jersey a court ruled that the city of Newark had to expand its programmatic accessibility as well by providing sign language interpreters at a municipal court wedding.[61]

Employment

Most employment-related cases have ended at the U.S. Circuit Court level, and many are settled out of court. In *Fredenburg v. Contra Costa County Dept. of Health Services,* 172 F. 3d 1176 (9th Cir. 1999), the court agreed that employees need not prove that they are qualified individuals with a disability to bring claims challenging the scope of medical examinations under the ADA. In another widely cited case, a policy that required an employee to be 100 percent healed before being allowed to return to work was deemed a per se violation of the ADA.[62]

Title I of the ADA does prohibit discrimination and appears to foster the goals of allowing individuals with disabilities to compete in the workplace, but it does not provide an entitlement to either cash or a job. It applies only to individuals who are "qualified," but it also requires employers to make appropriate adjustments to their workplaces so that a disabled person becomes more likely to be "qualified." Potential employees are given the right to demand "reasonable accommodations" to allow them to meet the "essential functions" of the job.[63] The result is a statute that

"draws upon the traditions of both civil rights laws as well as disability entitlement programs to create a complex, 'second generation' statute that aims
to achieve the negative liberty of self-sufficiency while fostering the positive right to accommodation."[64]

FUSION OF POSITIVE AND NEGATIVE RIGHTS

These individual cases do little to help explain the more esoteric arguments
that continue to bring disputes to the courts. One of the best explanations
for the current status of the law is provided by Patricia Illingworth and
Wendy E. Parmet, who praise the fact that the ADA melds positive and negative rights. "Like other civil rights statutes, the ADA broadly prohibits discrimination on the basis of disability. However . . . the ADA does not stop
with a guarantee of equal opportunity understood within a negative-rights
framework. The ADA does not simply say that individuals with mobility
impairments have the same rights as others to climb the stairs. . . . The ADA
gives individuals with disabilities the positive right to demand changes (and
contributions) from others, including private actors, to enable persons with
disabilities to become self-sufficient and participate more fully in public
life."[65]

The "rights" argument continues to serve as a platform for opponents
of the ADA, who believe that the statute is trying to do the impossible.
Critics rightly contend that not every person with a disability will be able
to find full-time employment, nor will they be able to accomplish feats
involving physical strength their body no longer possesses. One scholar
writes, "The discussion of the ADA and other policies never confronts the
question . . . as to the appropriate differences toward one individual who
loses a job through labor market contractions and an otherwise identical
individual who loses the same type of job as a result of an illness or
injury."[66]

Advocates for persons with disabilities seldom argue that the ADA is a
cure-all for unemployment, lack of affordable housing, social isolation,
or other problems faced by the population at large. They do believe, how-

ever, that the statute is the only way of starting to end patterns of discrimination that have persisted for decades, just as the 1964 Civil Rights
Act was a first step in that direction for people of color. Even persons with
disabilities are likely to admit that they do not expect decades of stereotypes to vanish overnight; if anything, they often talk of "another century
of struggle."

   In 1990, however, the policy window did open for a short time, allowing activists to move forward with a legislative agenda that might not have
gone forward had they waited another decade or so. Chapter 7 identifies
some of the issues that still must be addressed in that second century, as
well as the controversies that surround them.

CHAPTER 7

Life beyond the ADA: Policy Hot Buttons

It is difficult, yet important, to identify some of the issues that have become "hot buttons" in American disability policy since the passage of the ADA. Although the statute made at least a symbolic stab at protecting the rights of persons with disabilities and attempting to end discrimination, it also spawned discussion and protest. This chapter attempts to chronicle and explain some of the more inflammatory topics that have dominated the debate; it also recognizes that many more could have been included. It is hoped that this brief synopsis of some of the more highly publicized issues that affect many disabled persons will serve as a roadmap for twenty-first-century policymaking.

REPRODUCTIVE RIGHTS AND TECHNOLOGY

Although there are dozens of books related to issues associated with disability culture, only recently has there been a systematic attempt to explore the issues of sexuality and reproduction, from the scientific and phenomenological perspectives. Although these topics are sensitive for most of the population, they are especially so for persons with disabilities. What makes this issue compelling in a contemporary context is the fact that recent medical advances and changes in attitudes have provided a framework not only for studying but simply for talking about topics that affect us all.

Numerous hot-button topics come under the general categories of reproductive rights and reproductive technology: adoption, intimate relationships, parenting, prenatal/genetic counseling, infertility, sexual health and functioning, family relationships, pregnancy and delivery, and dysfunction.[1] The federal government made reproductive technology a policy priority when, in 1990, Congress authorized the $3 billion Human Genome Project to map the genes in human cells. The ultimate goal—to develop testing and treatment of the nearly 5,000 diseases that have a genetic basis—already is having a profound effect on prospective parents and health care professionals. With advances in medical procedures such as ultrasound, amniocentesis, and genetic testing, disability groups have warned that technology may become an enemy for persons with disabilities.[2] Yet from all indications, science is moving faster than the ethical debate, and policymaking is not keeping up.

For instance, a two-year study of the disability rights perspective on prenatal testing conducted by The Hastings Center (funded in part by the National Institute on Disability and Rehabilitation Research) found little consensus among biologists, physicians, ethicists, sociologists, and educators who participated.[3] Their concerns included a discussion of the "any/particular distinction," which refers to the difference between the decision to simply not have any child at all at the time (as with a woman who becomes pregnant who was not planning a family and decides to seek an abortion) and the decision to abort a particular fetus, even if the mother wants a child, because prenatal testing has revealed that the fetus has an impairment or deformity. The latter decision often leads to a selective abortion—when a pregnancy is planned but the fetus is perceived as having undesirable characteristics, such as Down Syndrome, spina bifida, cystic fibrosis, sickle cell anemia, or a similar birth defect.

The debate already is much more than an academic exercise. In November 2000 a French court ruled in favor of an eighteen-year-old boy, Nicholas Perruche, who sought compensation from his mother's doctor for having been born, in what has become known as a "wrongful life" case. The plaintiff's attorneys argued that a medical laboratory had failed to diagnose his mother's rubella and that the doctor did not advise her to have an abortion to prevent birth defects.[4] The family spent thirteen years in litigation on behalf of their son. France's highest court, Cour de Cassation, ordered that damages be paid to Perruche, who is partially blind and cannot speak or hear, as well as to his family. The boy is now in the care of a government institution. The ruling caused an uproar in France, with disability advocates arguing that the case was not only unethical but that it placed a price on human life because the court would set the level of damages. Antiabortion groups expressed the view that the ruling would reinforce the legal status of the unborn, even though similar cases brought by parents of disabled children have been thrown out by the court.

To date, U.S. courts have been unwilling to allow suits by a child against a parent, although there are some precedents in which a child has sued the mother's physician for failure to warn her of the potential risk that led to deformity. In 1984 the New Jersey Supreme Court allowed recovery of damages against a doctor sought by a child for "diminished childhood" because the child stated that she would rather not have been born than to have been born disabled.[5]

As Andrews and Hilbert note, "The very notion of wrongful birth and wrongful life—conveying the idea that having a child with a disability that could have been 'prevented' through abortion is some legal wrong—seems vastly at odds with the ideas about disability that serve as the foundation for the Americans with Disabilities Act. At the same time, however, some disability rights activists are strongly prochoice and feel uncomfortable restricting women's rights to terminate a pregnancy."[6] Disability advocates worry that courts will begin to find that physicians have a duty to offer prenatal tests and that women will be virtually forced to accept them.[7] Alabama law, for example, already defines as state policy "the prevention of birth defects and mental retardation through education, genetic counseling, and amniocentesis."[8]

The debate harkens back to the practice of eugenics discussed in chapter 2. It also reopens the definition of perceived normalcy and the concept that there is some type of agreed upon standard for which lives are worth living and which are not. It also highlights the fact that stereotypes about life with a disability or raising a disabled child still affect attitudes about abortion. A study conducted at Oregon's Health Sciences University asked pregnant women about their images of disability and their attitudes toward bearing a child with a disability. The results showed that although the women had very positive feelings and "almost romanticized attitudes" in general about people with disabilities, there was a dramatic difference when they were asked how they would feel if a child they bore had a disability; in the latter case, respondents were "fearful and negative." The results showed "a dynamic and somewhat confused mix of old images of mental retardation and incapacity juxtaposed with new images of different but 'special' children—and absolutely no way to sort them out."[9]

Over the past several years, the debate has become even more strident. Prenatal diagnosis, one researcher says, is "an assembly line approach to the products of conception separating out those we wish to develop from those we wish to discontinue."[10] The problem is exacerbated, some observers believe, by the fact that few people have contact with individuals with disabilities and consequently may overestimate their cost to society and underestimate their contribution to society. Physicians themselves may complicate decision making because even those who treat people with disabilities may have inaccurate impressions of the lives of such people if they interact with disabled persons only in a medical or treatment setting.[11]

Although the ADA was designed to prevent discrimination against persons with disabilities, it offers little legal protection when genetic technology is at issue. Almost half of the states currently recognize wrongful birth cases, with laws creating a duty on the part of doctors to offer genetic testing services to their high-risk patients. Physicians also can be sued for negligence if the mother is not told about the increased genetic risk and the availability of genetic testing such as amniocentesis.[12] Although society generally is in agreement that it is inappropriate to use genetic testing as an option in determining the sex of a fetus, the lines are less clear with regard to conditions that commonly are considered to be disabilities, especially when they are treatable.

The answer? Some scholars believe that wrongful death and wrongful life cases should be eliminated entirely as causes of action. If the ADA truly does eliminate discrimination and barriers encountered by persons with disabilities, such a move might make more sense. Yet at a time when the discrimination clearly remains pervasive for many disabled people, there probably is more support among activists for some type of line-drawing on the use of genetic testing. The politics-makes-strange-bedfellows alliance of disability rights activists and pro-life groups complicates the matter to some degree. To pro-life supporters for whom abortion is never an option, there is no need for thresholds or assessments on the quality of life. There is another reality, however, in which health care resources are being prioritized and rationed—a reality in which persons with disabilities may be placed lower on the priority list for treatment and care.[13] With those sorts of complications, reproductive technology policy becomes even more problematic.

Not Dead Yet

One of the most compelling and active elements in the disability rights movement is represented by Not Dead Yet (NDY), a group that is firmly opposed to any form of passive or active intervention in the process of dying. The terms "active" and "passive" commonly are used to distinguish between avoiding artificially prolonging the life of a terminally ill patient (passive) and the deliberate termination of life to avoid suffering (active euthanasia, or assisted suicide). For people with disabilities, the issue has become literally life-threatening. It also has a complex history that includes religious groups, medical practitioners, and zealots of various persuasions.[14]

The Euthanasia Society of America was established in 1938—the first formal organization in the emerging right-to-die movement in the United States. For the most part, however, the group was politically inactive for several decades because it received little support from the public or from political leaders. In the 1940s, with life extension made possible through advances in medical technology (including societal approval for harvesting human organs), social ethicists began to debate issues surrounding the prolongation of life. The Catholic Church entered the discussion in 1957 when Pope Pius XII differentiated between "ordinary" and "extraordinary" means of medical care—a move that is said to have given tacit permission to millions of Catholics to forego medical care that prolonged a painful existence.[15] In 1968 the World Medical Association confirmed its opposition to active euthanasia, as did the British Medical Association in 1969.

The debate in the United States became more strident in the late 1960s and 1970s with the publication of a series of books on euthanasia, including Elisabeth Kubler-Ross's *On Death and Dying*[16] and Glaser and Strauss's *Awareness of Dying*.[17] The public was further drawn into the issue through the highly publicized case of Karen Ann Quinlan—a young woman who was diagnosed as being in a persistent vegetative state and whose parents sought to have her removed from a respirator. Quinlan was not the only individual around whom the euthanasia debate was framed, however. In 1989 a Georgia court ruled that Larry McAfee had the "right" to be given a sedative and removed from the respirator that was keeping him alive. He later changed his mind, after meeting with disability rights advocates, as did Elizabeth Bouvia, a California woman who checked into a hospital and requested that physicians medicate her for pain while she starved herself to death.[18] In 1997, however, the U.S. Supreme Court ruled that there is no constitutional "right to die," leaving to the states the question of whether to legalize physician-assisted suicide (PAS).[19]

Several right-to-die organizations emerged in the 1980s and 1990s, partly as a result of passage of legislation in California that recognized a "living will" that allowed terminally ill individuals to make decisions about their own care. The Euthanasia Society branched out to become the Euthanasia Educational Fund; it was followed by the Society for the Right to Die and by Concern for Dying. In 1980 the World Federation of Right to Die Societies was established with twenty-seven groups from eighteen countries as the global debate expanded. That same year, the Society for the Right to Die and Concern for Dying merged under the name Choice in Dying; this development was followed by the establishment of the Hemlock Society. The latter group became the more controversial because it advocated active as well as passive euthanasia.[20] Its leader, Derek Humphry, served as a charismatic voice for the right-to-die movement, and his two major books, *Let Me Die Before I Wake*[21] and *Final Exit*,[22] brought the issue to the policy agenda more than ever before.

At the heart of the debate is the position of right-to-die advocates and groups such as the American Civil Liberties Union that requests from people seeking passive or active euthanasia are a reasonable response that should be humanely granted by members of the medical profession. Disability rights groups, in contrast, feel that such attitudes underscore a belief that life as a disabled person is no longer worth living. Disabled individuals' desire to end their lives, disability rights activists believe, stems more often from depression caused by isolation, lack of access to pain medication, or the sense that they have become a burden to their families and society.[23]

NDY emerged as a countermovement to PAS organizations in 1996. Its leaders, such as cofounder Diane Coleman, argue that disabled patients, who are already vulnerable and subject to discrimination, will be more likely to die if the euthanasia movement becomes more widespread. Their fears include the belief that disabled patients will be pressured to sign Do Not Resuscitate (DNR) orders or led to believe that they have an obligation to limit the costs of their care. Active euthanasia opponents also include members of the conservative right-to-life movement, who fear that the unborn also will become vulnerable. In opposing legalization of PAS, the countermovement's members have formed informal partnerships among various organizations. Their tactics have become more militant, including the takeover of the Colorado headquarters of the Hemlock Society in January 1998.[24]

NDY also has been active in protesting Oregon's PAS law—the first in the nation. The law sets forth specific circumstances under which PAS is legal: Terminally ill, mentally capable adult residents can get a prescription for a lethal dose of medicine from a physician if they make numerous oral and written requests within certain time periods and follow specific procedures. Physicians who assist such patients are held to a lengthy list of conditions and requirements.[25] The result, according to the *New England*

Journal of Medicine, is that during its first full year (1998), twenty-three persons (eighteen of whom had cancer) received prescriptions for lethal medication under the Oregon law. Of the twenty-three, fifteen died after taking the medication, another six died of their underlying illnesses, and two were still alive.[26] In 2001 the state's Health Division announced that twenty-seven more people used the law's provisions in the third year of the law's implementation—the same number as for 1999.[27]

Although these statistics rebut the predictions of NDY supporters that the Oregon law would open the floodgates of PAS, many observers believe that because of the U.S. Supreme Court's rulings in *Washington v. Glucksberg* and *Vacco v. Quill* and the controversial nature of the issue, PAS is not likely to spread rapidly as a solution to inadequate end-of-life care. In 1997 and 1998, bills on assisted suicide were introduced in twenty-six states. All were defeated. Voters in Michigan and Washington State rejected state ballot measures to legalize PAS, and several other states approved new bans on the practice.[28]

In California, an attempt to enact a "Death With Dignity" bill ended abruptly when the measure's sponsor met opposition from a coalition of disability organizations, advocates for poor people, consumer advocates, medical and hospice organizations, Catholic groups, and others. Members of the state legislature clearly did not want to see a vote on such a contentious issue during the 2000 electoral cycle, although the sponsor says she will reintroduce the bill.[29]

One of NDY's primary targets has been Dr. Jack Kevorkian, the Michigan pathologist who is either a savior or a murderer, depending on one's perspective. "Dr. Death," as he is commonly known, admits to assisting in more than 100 suicides since 1990. In 1996 the *British Medical Journal* declared Kevorkian "a hero," calling him "a man of action unmotivated by greed or fame, and who is not afraid of criticism or of prosecution. Kevorkian did not stop at words. He acted to end what he perceived as suffering and then turned to the law and said 'I dare you to stop me.'"[30] Kevorkian now sits in a prison cell after being convicted of second-degree murder of a patient in violation of a 1998 Michigan law that outlawed PAS.

His actions were documented in a videotape aired on television's *60 Minutes* that showed him injecting a terminally ill man with a fatal dose of potassium chloride, in a direct challenge to prosecutors to arrest and charge him—which they did.

Members of NDY may have thought that in going to prison, Kevorkian had been silenced. That was somewhat true until April 10, 2000, when the Gleitsman Foundation honored Kevorkian with its Citizen Activist Award in ceremonies at Harvard University, giving Kevorkian some semblance of credibility. In response to NDY's protest of the award, some members of the award committee (which includes actor Ted Danson, Marian Wright Edelman of the Children's Defense Fund, and feminist activist Gloria Steinem) expressed some displeasure at the selection but did not withdraw the honor.[31]

NDY members also have targeted Dr. Peter Singer, who was appointed to the Ira W. DeCamp professorship at Princeton University's Center for Human Values in 1998. Singer, whom the group considers "much more dangerous than Kevorkian,"[32] is best known as an animal rights activist. He also has spoken out, however, in favor of the right of a parent to kill a disabled child, and he has been perceived as taking an openly antidisability stance. His hiring, critics argue, would never have happened if his views were racist or sexist, exemplary of the marginalization of disability as a type of discrimination.[33] NDY members held protests at Princeton to draw attention to Singer's belief that parents should be allowed to kill infants younger than twenty-eight days if they want to try again for a "better" child. The protests led to a controversial debate in 1999 in which Singer said that the NDY protestors were not happy to be disabled and would certainly opt to be cured if cures were available. "Of course they would," he said.[34]

JERRY'S KIDS AND TELETHONS

It may have started out innocently enough: During the 1930s, various charities used posters portraying children as a way of raising funds to address illnesses such as polio, cerebral palsy, and muscular dystrophy. The poster children considered it an honor to represent their peers, and the results inevitably brought in money from people touched by the sight of a disabled child. In the 1950s television raised the financial stakes through the sponsorship of telethons, the most famous of which was promoted by comedian Jerry Lewis on behalf of people with muscular dystrophy. Unlike the silent faces on the posters, the children and parents on the MD Association telethons were on live television, recounting lives of sadness and dreams of cures. The money, viewers were told, went to services but primarily was spent on the search for a cure.

In the 1970s, as the disability rights movement began to grow, protests erupted against the use of telethons as a fundraising technique. Previous poster children formed an organization called Jerry's Orphans, criticizing what they believe to be the exploitation of disabled persons. The group began to demonstrate against the Jerry Lewis telethon in 1991, and local activists now protest against local television stations that carry the annual Labor Day broadcast. United Cerebral Palsy Association telethons in New York were picketed in 1976 and 1977 by the group Disabled In Action. Its members called the programs demeaning and paternalistic shows that celebrate and encourage pity.

As director of the Disability Rights Center, Evan Kemp, Jr., criticized the MD telethon in a 1981 *New York Times* editorial, arguing that the program reinforces a stigma against disabled people.[35] Jerry Lewis was so angered by Kemp's words that he launched a public campaign against Kemp in retaliation, attempting in 1990 to get President George Bush to fire the outspoken advocate from his position as chair of the Equal Employment Opportunity Commission. Kemp's current website includes a lengthy story that calls Lewis a "pity mongering patron" with a notoriously explosive personality and admitted ties to organized crime.[36]

Additional criticism has focused on Lewis himself. The two-day telethon, which includes scenes from Broadway musicals, celebrities, and local talent, goes on through the night, with Lewis becoming increasingly exhausted. One viewer notes that in 1974 or 1975, he watched the show in the early morning hours as Lewis rambled on about his motivation for the telethon. "My recollection is that he says something like, 'They ask me why I do it. Well, maybe I'll say someday. However, they're going to have to come across with the big bucks before I tell this story. Then maybe I'll say.' In hindsight and after hearing revelations concerning Mr. Lewis's prescription drug addiction during that era, I have always wondered how chemically enhanced the moment was."[37]

Others believe Lewis is dangerously out of touch, especially after he wrote a cover story for *Parade* magazine that referred to disabled people as "cripples" and called dystrophic illness "the curse that attacks children of all ages."[38] After putting himself in a wheelchair to feel what it might be like, he wrote further that he felt "trapped and suffocated." "I realize my life is half, so I must learn to do things halfway. I may be a full human being in my heart and soul, yet I am still half a person."[39]

In 2001 Lewis announced that he would cut back on the number of hours he spent hosting the annual Labor Day Telethon, due to illness. Activists countered, however, that Lewis took the action in response to a CBS News correspondent's questions about protestors. Lewis said, "I'm telling people about a child in trouble! If it's pity, we'll get some money. I'm just giving you the facts!. . . Pity? [If] you don't want to be pitied because you're a cripple in a wheelchair, stay in ya house!" The MDA later issued an apology, as did Lewis.[40]

Such comments outrage disability advocates such as Carol Gill, who responded, "My wheelchair isn't an imprisonment—it's a tremendous vehicle of liberation. What's a steel imprisonment is those negative images that Jerry Lewis and the MDA promote. The stereotypes keep us locked in a cell of discrimination and prejudice."[41]

CHRISTOPHER REEVE AND THE MYTH OF THE SUPERCRIP

Although Jack Kevorkian undoubtedly is one of the most despised and cursed individuals by many disability rights activists, he shares that distinction with Christopher Reeve, the actor best known for his portrayal of Superman. In 1995 Reeve was riding in a charity equestrian event and injured his spinal cord in an accident. His resulting quadriplegia and celebrity status brought him instantaneous worldwide attention, not only because of his injuries but because of his response to them. Speaking to the Democratic National Convention from his motorized wheelchair in 1996, Reeve briefly mentioned the Americans with Disabilities Act but focused on the need for increased funding to find a cure for spinal cord injuries.

Among mainstream activists, Reeve is publicly and privately sanctioned because of his emphasis on finding a cure and because of his belief that living with a disability is a fate worse than death.[42] In an interview with Barbara Walters on the television program *20/20* in 1996, Reeve told the public that he had briefly thought of suicide after his accident because he thought living "wasn't worth everybody's trouble." In another interview with *Time* magazine's Roger Rosenblatt, he said, "When they told me what my condition was, I felt that I was no longer a human being. . . . Maybe this just isn't worth it. Maybe I should just check out."[43]

The "cure mentality" has angered so many activists within the disability community. They believe that Reeve's approach simplifies a complex issue, making it seem as if all one has to do is wait for medical science to make everything in their lives perfect—that disabilities can be "fixed" just as someone would fix a broken toaster. In the meantime, issues such as accessibility and discrimination are tabled while vast funds are raised for conditions that may never be curable.

"I'm not that interested in lower sidewalks and better wheelchairs," Reeve says. "It's nice to have good equipment and access while you're disabled, but I think all of us with these problems should be allowed to regard them as a temporary setback rather than a way of life."[44] Such comments anger activists in the disability rights movement who have worked so long and hard for legal protections such as the ADA.

In online chat rooms, the comments become even more inflammatory and angry. Activist and researcher Phyllis Rubenfeld notes, "I'm sorry that you can't see that Christopher Reeve is setting us back a zillion years." Another responds, "Reeve has been able to give visibility to the insurance problems, medical costs, etc. of SCI [spinal cord injuries] to policymakers. Not many changes have occurred yet but it is a strong voice." And one website played the theme from the movie "Superman" in the background and asked visitors to vote on whether Reeve is a "humanitarian, superman, or selfish bastard."

Some activists were indignant when Reeve was named to the board of directors of the National Organization on Disability (NOD) in 1997. The organization, which is cross-disability oriented and receives no government funding, relies entirely on donations from the private sector. Reeve also is chairman of the board of the American Paralysis Association and president of the Christopher Reeve Foundation. There is little doubt among his detractors that Reeve represents the kind of celebrity fundraiser that has become the mainstay for other medical conditions such as AIDS and Parkinson's disease. In making the announcement of Reeve's appointment, NOD President Alan A. Reich commented, "Thanks to Christopher, the field is attracting more funding and more scientific investigation by neuroscientists."[45]

Some detractors, however, feel that celebrity disease lobbyists are focusing attention on issues in health policy out of proportion to their statistical significance. In 1998, for instance, AIDS and breast cancer were reported to have received $2,400 per patient and $230 per patient in research tax dollars, respectively, compared with $28 per patient for diabetes—even though diabetes killed more people in 1997 than AIDS and breast cancer combined.[46]

There is no argument that every death from disease is a tragedy. Individuals who advocate for specific illnesses or conditions, such as Reeve, are criticized for trying to drive public health research funding by public relations. One conservative columnist noted, "Instead of hyping the risks of fashionable illnesses embraced by Hollywood, report on the realities of the world's mundane health threats, such as diarrhea, which kills an estimated 1 million children worldwide every year."[47]

DEAF CULTURE AND COCHLEAR IMPLANTS

Writer Joseph Shapiro notes that in American Sign Language (ASL), "to say that someone is 'very hard of hearing' means the opposite of its definition in English. To deaf people, to have no hearing is the standard. To be " 'very hard of hearing' is to deviate greatly from the standard, or to hear quite well."[48]

Sign language has been used in various forms throughout history, often in religious orders whose devotees adopted a vow of silence. In the mid-fifteenth century, Benedictine monks used sign language as a teaching tool for deaf children. Two centuries later, the French had developed a more comprehensive version that was used by the Abbe Charles Michel de l'Epee in Paris.[49] When Thomas Gallaudet visited Europe in 1815, he learned to blend the French language into an American version that was introduced to the American School for the Deaf by his colleague Laurent Clerc in 1817. By the 1860s, however, sign language was being replaced by "oralism"— the use of speech and lip reading.[50]

ASL did not return to favor until 1960, when linguists began to study what at the time was considered an esoteric language with little meaning for deaf people.[51] Now there is general agreement that it is a complex, visual-spatial language that bears no grammatical similarities to English. ASL is not merely gestural because it also uses facial features and the use of space surrounding the signer to describe places and persons who are not present. Although sign languages develop specific to their community and are not universal, ASL is now the fourth most commonly used language in the United States.[52]

In the mid-1980s, the deaf community began to coalesce and, in some ways, become more visible. Actress Marlee Matlin won an Academy Award in 1986 (the first deaf actor to win an Oscar) for her portrayal of a deaf woman in the movie *Children of a Lesser God,* and she has played speaking and nonspeaking roles in other plays, movies, and television programs, including the popular series *The West Wing.*[53] Many Americans assume that all deaf persons use ASL to communicate, just as many assume all blind persons can read Braille.

Integration of deaf persons into mainstream society was not universally embraced, and some disability activists had a strong desire to be distinct and in some ways isolated from the hearing world. Separation of deaf people from others is not a new concept. From 1830 to 1900, the U.S. Bureau

of the Census included deaf persons in the category of "defectives." In the
1850s John Flournoy, a deaf activist, sought congressional approval for a
parcel of unsettled land and proposed the creation of a new state that
would be known as Gesturia, populated only by people who were deaf.
Also known as Deaf Mutia, the state would acknowledge the oppression
faced by persons who were deaf or hard of hearing. Deaf scholars, among
others, thought the plan was too ambitious, comparing it to the struggle
of the Mormons who moved to and settled in Utah. Some proposed an
alternative "deaf township."[54]

The goal of activists who have sought separation from not only the mainstream but from other persons with disabilities is the idea that deafness is
not a disability at all but the defining characteristic of a specific, identifiable
ethnic and linguistic minority. In 1972 linguist James Woodward argued that
a distinction needed to be made between persons who were considered deaf
because their hearing was impaired and deaf people who shared a common
language (ASL) and an identifiable culture. The term "deaf" has come to be
used as a way of defining individuals as members of a group who accept and
appreciate their uniqueness.[55] The study of deaf culture involves ethnogra-
phers, sociologists, linguists, political scientists, and other academic disciplines, yet even the term itself is not universally accepted. The use of the
uppercase term "Deaf" is now used to refer to people who self-identify
themselves as part of a culture, whereas the lower-case "deaf" is applied to
those with some form of audiological impairment.[56]

The concept of deaf culture also has its detractors, however. Some compare the desire to be separate from the rest of society to the integrationist
argument among black people. Frank Bowe, a leading deaf activist, believes
that the emphasis on separatism can cut deaf people off from the benefits
of the disability rights movement. From a different perspective, Robert
Funk, who has supported integration as a way of bringing more people with
disabilities into society, believes that "disability will disappear as an issue"
once businesses accommodate workers with disabilities, architects embrace
universal design, and buildings are made accessible to all persons.[57]

Deaf self-identity was challenged in 1985 when the U.S. Food and Drug
Administration approved for use an implant device that would be surgi-

cally inserted into a deaf person's cochlea, allowing the individual to hear. The implant is designed to bypass a damaged cochlea to stimulate the nerve fibers, at a cost of approximately $25,000. To some people the new technology was a miracle, allowing those who had been deaf for years to hear.[58] In 1995 the National Institutes of Health published a *Health Consensus Development Conference Statement* that concluded that cochlear implantation "improves communication ability in most adults with deafness and frequently leads to positive psychological and social benefits as well." The report indicated that children at least two years old and adults with profound deafness are the best candidates for implantation, although auditory performance varies among individuals.[59]

This "technological cure" has become perhaps one of the most contentious issues in Deaf life and medicine, especially among activists who believe the cochlear implant is a conspiracy designed to bring about the "genocide of deaf culture."[60] Some Deaf children believe it represents parental rejection and denial of their condition, especially when the child is born to hearing parents. "Because hearing parents 'can't find a place of acceptance' for their deaf children, they opt for the cochlear implant without exploring the possibilities of immersing them in the 'deaf culture,'" one Deaf activist writes. "They try to fix them."[61] Others have said that the procedure amounts to "another signal from hearing society that deaf people are simply not good enough as they are."[62] This latter sentiment appears to have split Deaf persons into opposite camps.

Owen Wrigley, who writes on the issue of identity formation, calls the development of the cochlear implant (and its successor, brain stem implants) forms of "deferments." He notes, "Technical and medical options aimed at reproducing speech and hearing are products of deferring. Technologies, be they tactile aids, implants, manual codes, or any technical mediation (including mainstreaming), all promise great potential, but that potential can only be realized after further 'development.' What is actually delivered, along with promises and pious exhortations, is but a small part of what was promised."[63]

The issue garnered media exposure when the documentary film *Sound and Fury* was released in theaters nationwide in October 2000. The film portrays a bitter debate among family members over whether to accept a cochlear implant for their child, arguing whether potential adverse effects would result in more harm than good. The National Association of the Deaf (NAD), responding to public and media interest, issued a position statement on cochlear implants about the time the film was released. The organization "recognizes that diversity within the deaf community itself, and within the deaf experience, has not been acknowledged or explained very clearly in the public forum. . . . Diversity requires mutual respect for individual and/or group differences and choices."[64]

The statement goes on to note that the NAD "recognizes the rights of parents to make informed choices for their deaf and hard of hearing children, respects their choice to use cochlear implants and all other assistive devices, and strongly supports the development of the whole child and of language and literacy. . . . While there are some successes with implants, success stories should not be over-generalized to every individual."[65]

This faint praise highlights the debate within the medical community among those who argue that deafness needs to be "fixed" in some way as well as among members of the deaf community who function well in both the hearing and deaf worlds. As one advocate writes, "If only the general public knew the inherent intelligence, brightness and rhythm within our world! We share a responsibility to educate others about our culture, language, and heritage."[66]

THE INTEGRATION MANDATE

Until the late 1990s, many disability activists believed that although the ADA was not universally implemented and enforced, it was relatively safe from legal challenge. It had received bipartisan congressional support and had been enacted and signed during a Republican administration. Although there is no doubt that the statute was in need of clarification on key points such as "reasonable accommodations" and "undue hardship," few observers expected that one of the decade's most important U.S. Supreme Court cases would challenge the concept of bringing an end to unnecessary segregation.

All that changed in 1998 when the state of Georgia petitioned the Supreme Court, asking the justices to hear its appeal of an 11th Circuit Court of Appeals ruling in *Olmstead v. L.C.* The case involved two women with mental disabilities who had voluntarily been admitted to the Georgia Regional Hospital in Atlanta and confined to the psychiatric unit. Although the treatment staff concluded that the two women could be cared for appropriately in a community-based program, the state refused to do so, citing inadequate funding. Initially, twenty-two states (along with the National Conference of State Legislatures) signed *amici* briefs in support of Georgia's position, but a well-orchestrated campaign by disability rights groups eventually led to a victory for people confined to institutions.

At the heart of the case was whether the state had unnecessarily discriminated against the two women on the basis of their disabilities, in violation of the ADA, by failing to provide the plaintiffs with care in the most integrated setting appropriate to their needs. The lower court's ruling set off a firestorm of debate over whether people who are unnecessarily institutionalized in state hospitals, nursing homes, and other state facilities have the right to receive appropriate treatment, including personal assistance services in their homes or other settings.

Under the administration of George Bush, the federal government had endorsed the principle of integration of people with disabilities into the wider population. In 1991 the Attorney General's office issued regulations stating that services or programs were to be offered in the most integrated setting appropriate to the needs of the disabled person—a regulation that came to be known as the "integration mandate." The appeals court had ruled that state budgetary restrictions were not a defense unless the cost of compliance was "so unreasonable given the demands of the state's mental health budget that it would fundamentally alter the service it provides."[67]

A coalition of groups led by ADAPT slowly began to turn public opinion against states that had signed on as *amici* to Georgia's petition. Calling the case "our *Brown v. Board of Education*," ADAPT's Campaign for Real Choice likened the case to that of Dred Scott, in which the Supreme Court ruled that a slave could not sue for his freedom.[68] ADAPT called on other disability, aging, family, and advocacy groups to organize a six-month statewide strategy against the states that had joined Georgia in the belief that their *amici* briefs had convinced the U.S. Supreme Court to hear the case.

The concerted effort by a coalition of groups to change the minds of state officials began to work. One by one, state attorneys general began to withdraw their support. Michigan's Solicitor General Thomas Casey had a change of heart, noting that after taking a "fresh look" at the case, his state had concluded that "Georgia's arguments are not consistent with the state of Michigan's position as a leader in community-based mental health care."[69] Massachusetts, Minnesota, and Louisiana withdrew their support after signing the final brief, and Alabama, California, Delaware, Florida, Maryland, Michigan, Nebraska, New Hampshire, Pennsylvania, South Dakota, Utah, and West Virginia declined to sign after initially supporting Georgia. Ten states continued to support Georgia's case: Colorado, Hawaii, Indiana, Mississippi, Montana, Nevada, South Carolina, Tennessee, Texas, and Wyoming.

The strategy demonstrated one of the few ways in which an interest group can affect the outcome of a case once it reaches the judicial arena. Because the justices are virtually isolated from any external political debate, putting pressure on the states to withdraw their support was a key tactic. By reducing the number of *amici* briefs filed in support of Georgia, advocates for disabled persons may have had an impact on the salience of the state's case.

Although U.S. Secretary of Health and Human Services Donna Shalala wrote the nation's governors that "unnecessary institutionalization of individuals with disabilities is discrimination under the Americans with Disabilities Act" and that "no person should have to live in a nursing home or other institution," progress on implementing *Olmstead* has been slow. ADAPT's leaders have placed the blame on the way the nation funds services and on a powerful nursing home lobby. The group has supported legislation that would allow persons who get Medicaid money to make a choice about where they wanted to get services (a topic discussed in more depth in chapter 8).[70]

Although some states—such as Missouri, Texas, Mississippi, Ohio, and Wisconsin—have moved toward plans that allow Medicaid funds to "follow the person," other states appear to need prodding to implement the integration mandate. In Louisiana, a class-action suit was filed in April 2000 over the state's long waiting list for home and community-based services and the lack of notification to disabled persons about their options. A similar suit was filed in Indiana by the Everybody Counts Center for Independent Living, charging that people are being inappropriately institutionalized.

The most comprehensive analysis of the *Olmstead* decision's implementation was conducted in 2001–2002 by the National Conference of State Legislatures, which conducted a fifty-state survey. The study found that 80 percent of the states have task forces, commissions, or state agency work groups to assess current long-term care systems and that many were developing plans. Ten states did not have an equivalent body. Eighteen states had issued plans or significant papers, with some states in the planning process. More important, perhaps, are the recommendations of the state commissions and their perceptions about major issues associated with implementation:

- Most states cited a lack of affordable and accessible housing and transportation as major barriers to serving more people in the community.
- There is a need for a coherent system to identify how many people with disabilities are currently institutionalized who are eligible for services.
- There is a severe shortage of long-term care workers who are qualified to provide more home- and community-based services.
- Most commissions did not think many sweeping reforms could happen without education for consumers, providers, and state agency officials.
- Assistance is needed in helping individuals make the transition from institutions into the community, including permanency planning for children currently residing in institutions.
- Expansion of Medicaid waiver programs is needed.

Calling the pace of implementation "slow," the study commented on the frustration being experienced by disability advocates, state officials, and other stakeholders. State budget shortfalls and declining state revenues, along with terrorism and state safety issues, are likely to delay implementation even further, the report concludes. "The short-term effects of the decision have not been dramatic on the care settings for people with disabilities. . . . The most important effect thus far is that it has caused providers, consumers, and state officials from various departments to jointly discuss long-term care reforms. . . . State plans are a work in progress that will evolve in response to funding, state input, agency-related initiatives, and continued growth and demand for community services and supports for people with disabilities."[71]

Meanwhile, Lois Curtis and Elaine Wilson—the two women identified only by their initials in the *Olmstead* case—have been guaranteed that they will be able to live in community-based housing for the rest of their lives. That guarantee was provided by Atlanta judge Marvin Shoob in July 2000 as part of a settlement agreement that resulted from the U.S. Supreme Court decision. Wilson had told the judge, "When I was in the hospital, I felt like I was in a little box." When she was told she would no longer be forced to live in an institution, Wilson responded, "I love my freedom."[72]

VIOLENCE AGAINST PEOPLE WITH DISABILITIES

One of the more recent issues that has made its way onto the policy agenda deals with violence against persons with disabilities, some of which has been linked to the growing problem of hate crimes (or bias crimes, as they also are known). One of the galvanizing events that ignited concern around the country was the highly publicized Glen Ridge case in New Jersey in March 1989. A seventeen-year-old woman with an IQ of 49 and a second grader's performance skills was lured into a basement recreation room by a group of high school senior athletes. They promised her that if she accompanied them, they would arrange a date for her with another boy she idolized. Instead, they repeatedly raped her with a broomstick, a baseball bat, and another stick while their friends cheered; no one intervened. The following day, a group of thirty boys tried to get her to go back to the basement with them, and she refused.

The gang rape highlighted what many advocates considered stereotypical treatment of disabled persons by law enforcement agencies and a criminal justice system that refuses to take such attacks seriously. Bernard Lefkowitz, who has written one of the most moving books about the incident, found it difficult to understand why the Glen Ridge community was so supportive of the young men—raising $30,000 to defray their legal bills and referring to the young woman as a slut. The superintendent of schools, a woman, urged the school to "stand by our boys."[73]

The defense attorneys argued that the young woman had provoked and enjoyed the assault; prosecutor Robert Laurino maintained that the nature of her disability did not allow her to give informed consent. The press noted that the victim previously had consensual sexual relations and that she had willingly followed the young men to the basement room. Witnesses for the prosecution, however, pointed out that such behavior, including a desire to please and comply, often is part of the training and treatment of mentally retarded people, making them more vulnerable. In this case, the victim had been taunted and manipulated by her classmates for more than a decade. Finally an athlete who had heard about what had taken place told a teacher what he knew; at his graduation ceremony a few weeks later, the audience shouted that he was a snitch for breaking the code of silence among his athletic clique. Many of the students wore yellow ribbons at the event, saying they were in memory of the four young men who had been arrested and were not allowed to attend the graduation ceremony. As Lefkowitz sees it, "This was their way of recognizing these young men and proclaiming their loyalty to them."[74]

In March 1993, three of the defendants were convicted of sexual assault and conspiracy, and a fourth was convicted of conspiracy. All four went free while the convictions were appealed to the New Jersey appellate court in 1997, which overturned a part of the convictions on the ground that there was insufficient evidence of coercion. The assailants were then convicted of having sex with "a mentally defective person" and went on with their lives.[75]

The Glen Ridge case is only one incident in the nation's history of hate, discrimination, and violence. When the Ku Klux Klan was active in the late nineteenth century, various states enacted laws to address bias-related crimes, primarily against blacks. The laws referenced the wearing of hoods, burning of crosses, desecration of religious buildings, and interruption of religious observances. These laws were followed in the 1950s by calls from the civil rights movement for more protection against violent discriminatory acts.

In the early 1990s Congress passed a series of statutes in response to acts of bias-related violence around the nation. When violence is motivated by prejudice because of a person's characteristics—including race, religion, ethnic background, national origin, gender, or sexual orientation—the crime is considered to be not only against the individual but also an assault against an entire group of people. Proponents of hate crimes legislation argue that bias crimes must be afforded special attention because the state has a compelling interest in protecting the community.[76] Persons with disabilities rarely have been covered by these statutes, however.

The federal government and the states have taken a wide variety of legislative approaches to bias crime. The purpose is threefold: to protect the rights of individuals to be free from random violence against their person or property; to deter people from acting on their biases; and to punish violent behavior. Hate crimes statutes serve as a statement of abhorrence of all forms of violence that is motivated by prejudice, regardless of the object of that prejudice.[77] The 1990 Hate Crimes Statistics Act was the first of a series of laws, initially attempting to establish a nationwide system for tracking bias crime statistics. Several states also enacted legislation to train law enforcement officers to recognize hate crimes and report them. In 1994 federal legislation was enacted to enhance sentencing standards for defendants who were found guilty of hate crimes, and in 1996 Congress turned to the issue of arson involving churches. President Clinton convened the first-ever White House Conference on Hate Crimes in November 1997, but the one-day event did not include crimes against disabled persons.

Under a different type of statute—the 1994 Violent Crime and Law Enforcement Act—Congress included disability as a distinct category, defining a hate crime as one in which "the defendant intentionally selects a victim, or in the case of a property crime, the property that is the object of the crime, because of the actual or perceived race, color, national origin, ethnicity, gender, disability, or sexual orientation of any person."[78] Recognizing that existing laws were not sufficient in protecting these classifications, members of Congress introduced—but were unsuccessful in gaining passage of—Hate Crime Prevention Acts in 1998 and again in 2000. The proposed statutes broadened protection by including crimes that were based on sexual orientation, gender, or disability. Funds also were to be made available for technical assistance, research, and provision of victim services. Disability rights advocates also were unsuccessful in securing support for the Crime Victims with Disabilities Awareness Act in 1998. The measure would have provided less than $1 million to include disability as a category in the National Crime Victims Survey and increased public awareness of the issue.

Some observers refer to persons with disabilities who are the victims of physical abuse, violence, or intimidation as the "invisible victims." Their exact numbers are unknown because many crimes against disabled people are not separately categorized or, more commonly, are unreported or never prosecuted. One study published by the Institute on Community Integration at the University of Minnesota noted that the rates of violent crime against people with developmental or other severe disabilities are four to ten or more times higher than the rate against the general population. Another study reported that 83 percent of women and 32 percent of men with developmental disabilities in the sample had been sexually assaulted;[79] other researchers have found that of those who were sexually assaulted, half had been assaulted ten or more times.[80]

One advocate who was among the first to document and speak out against this type of violence is Barbara Faye Waxman, who believes that people with disabilities face a pattern of oppressive social treatment and hatred. Waxman likens hate crimes against people with disabilities to the misogyny faced by women, homophobia against gay men and lesbians, anti-Semitism against Jews, and racism against people of color. She includes in her definition of hate crimes against disabled people the vandalizing and firebombing of community-based group homes for developmentally disabled adults, attacks on people who are mentally retarded, and vandalism of assistive devices such as wheelchairs or van lifts.[81] Other reports have found that crimes against persons with disabilities often are extremely violent and calculated to injure, control, and humiliate the victim. Waxman believes such attacks are consequences of segregation and poverty and the dependence of persons with disabilities on others, which makes them easier targets.[82]

There is another disturbing perspective that argues that antidiscrimination laws have tended to rotate around a single-axis framework. Kimberle Crenshaw writes that color obliterates gender and thus race eclipses disability, thereby marginalizing people who do not fit clearly into a recognized minority status—what legal theorists call intersectionality. The result is that many individuals, including disabled people, are edited out of civil rights and employment decisions, which tend to focus more on the issue of race.[83] Thus, adds Lennard Davis, "when disability meets race, disability is propelled to the margins of the class."[84]

The Washington, D.C.-based Center for Women Policy Studies has developed ten recommendations for the Attorney General related to violence against persons with disabilities, especially women. The effort includes studies and a report to Congress on the need for an improved data collection system, information on how well agencies that receive funding for crime victims programs are complying with the ADA, the training needs of police officers to identify and investigate violence against disabled women and girls, and the training needs of judges who hear such cases.[85]

Invisible Disabilities

A blue wheelchair is the universal symbol for disability, and many individuals assume that it refers primarily to a person's lack of mobility.

Millions of other people, however, have "invisible disabilities" that result in pervasive stigma, discrimination, and stereotypes. Based on the number of charges filed with the EEOC involving emotional or psychiatric impairment during the period from 1992 to 1996, these cases involve nearly 13 percent of all claims.[86]

Invisible disabilities cover a wide range of conditions and illnesses. One website index lists impairments including brain injury, chronic fatigue syndrome, deafness and hearing loss, diabetes, epilepsy, fetal alcohol syndrome, narcolepsy, and repetitive stress injuries. Perhaps the largest category under the ADA, however, is psychiatric disabilities, which the EEOC has interpreted to mean a mental impairment that includes major depression, bipolar disorder, anxiety disorders, schizophrenia, and personality disorders. To be classified as a "disability," the impairment also must substantially limit one or more life activities of the individual. The substantial limitation language means that an individual is assessed in terms of the severity of the limitation and the length of time it restricts a major life activity.[87]

One of the most controversial aspects of the EEOC's guidelines is whether the corrective effects of medications can be considered in deciding if an impairment is so severe that it substantially limits a major life activity. In three 1999 cases involving physical impairments, the U.S. Supreme Court ruled that under the ADA, if a person has little or no difficulty performing a major life activity because of the use of a mitigating measure, then the person does not meet the criteria for being defined as "disabled." Despite those rulings, the EEOC maintains that the legislative history of the ADA makes clear that medications would not be considered as mitigating measures in cases of mental impairment. The interpretation of mental impairment also includes chronic, episodic disorders, such as major depression.[88]

Although the legal interpretations present some hurdles for persons with psychiatric illnesses, even more difficult are decisions about disclosure of their disability, particularly to an employer or potential employer. The rules implementing the ADA clearly state that a job application cannot ask questions about emotional illness or psychiatric disability, except in very limited circumstances after an offer of employment has been made. At that point, the employer may require a medical or psychiatric exam if it relates to the disability and may ask questions about the need for reasonable accommodations. That request need not be made at the beginning of employment and may be made by a surrogate, such as a health professional or family member.

Reasonable accommodations for persons with psychiatric illnesses can pose unique challenges for employers, especially because they must be addressed on an ad hoc basis. For example, an individual who needs time off from work to obtain treatment might be allowed to use any accrued paid leave or additional unpaid leave, as long as the person's absence does not create an undue hardship on the employer's business. Similarly, hiring a job coach to help train a person with a disability is considered reasonable, as is a modified work schedule. The law does allow an employer to exclude an individual from employment, however, if the individual poses a direct threat for safety reasons; this provision applies in situations in which the individual's or others' safety is at high risk.[89]

In several situations, the EEOC has made clear that it disagrees with the courts' rulings on whether the use of mitigating medications precludes an individual from being defined as disabled. The commission also has expressed its frustration with cases that deal with a request for accommodation. The EEOC uses language such as "incorrectly decided" when it refers to rulings with which it disagrees—such as a 1995 case in which an employer refused to honor a family member's request for accommodation. The court held that the employer had not been alerted to the employee's disability even though the employee's sister phoned the employer repeatedly, informing the company that the employee was falling apart mentally and that the family was trying to get her into a hospital.[90] These are major policy arguments that have yet to be settled and could have a substantial impact on persons covered by the ADA.

A second category of invisible illnesses that has attracted considerable public attention is multiple chemical sensitivity, or MCS. Also referred to as "environmental illnesses," MCS represents an allergic-type response to commonly used synthetic substances, including pesticides, detergents, and perfumes. MCS is said to affect 15–30 percent of Americans to one degree or another, with symptoms such as headaches, fatigue, depression, and respiratory problems. After a time, even low-level exposure may cause symptoms, frequently affecting an individual's overall physical and emotional health. Causes of the sensitivity are thought to include substances (paints and solvents, insect repellant, cleaning supplies, mercury amalgam fillings in teeth, Agent Orange), and processes (offgassing of adhesives used in installing new carpets, lack of adequate building ventilation).[91] Several other invisible yet disabling conditions, such as fibromyalgia and chronic fatigue syndrome, also are believed to be associated with MCS.

A multitude of organizations provide information and support to persons with environmental illnesses, such as the National Center for Environmental Health Strategies, the National Coalition for the Chemically Injured, and the Environmental Health Network. In 1965 a group of clinicians devoted to management and prevention of environmentally triggered illnesses formed the American Academy of Environmental Medicine. Several communities have been built in the southwest United States that utilize "safe" building materials and eliminate the use of products that are thought to exacerbate symptoms. Other individuals who have been affected live in homemade tents or trailers, moving frequently as they become sensitized to the local area. In San Rafael, California, a specially designed, eleven-unit apartment building was opened in 1994; it was constructed and maintained to reduce the toxic load on residents. The builders of Ecology House estimate that about 11 percent of the complex's $1.8 million development cost is attributable to the extra cost of special features to accommodate persons with MCS.[92]

Policy responses to environmental illnesses have varied considerably, although the primary focus has been on research. In 1996 a National Academy of Sciences report targeted six categories of chemicals that should be given high priority for neurotoxicity testing: fragrances, insecticides, heavy metals, solvents, food additives, and certain air pollutants. Two years later, the federal Agency for Toxic Substances and Disease Registry issued a 100-page draft report on MCS that was criticized heavily by disability advocates. They argued that the report had been written by persons with a conflict of interest that had not been disclosed, that it represented a limited sample of medical literature and agency experience with MCS, and that one of its principal authors was an employee of the Environmental Sensitivities Research Institute (allegedly funded by the chemical and pesticide industries).[93] At the local level, several groups have lobbied to restrict the use of fragrance products, especially in public places. The San Francisco chapter of the Sierra Club, for example, issued a 1998 resolution that called for education about "the insidious nature of toxic chemical fragrance products and their role in associated illnesses and disabilities for both users and secondhand recipients alike."[94] Several cities now issue statements requesting that the use of personal fragrances be limited in attending public functions.

Some people believe that the term "invisible disability" is a misnomer, simply because it assumes that there is a difference between the barriers people with such disabilities face and those encountered by those with a "visible" disability. The latter category includes individuals who use wheelchairs, canes, hearing aids, crutches, walkers, and service animals. Persons with environmental or chronic illnesses who "do not look sick" often are accused, however, of faking or imagining their disability. There are no assistive devices that can help them when the illness is triggered by secondhand tobacco smoke, no barriers to make more accessible when the person is HIV-positive. Although the categorization of disabilities may seem divisive, it also points to the individualization of disabilities and the realization that there is nothing wrong with a disability that is somehow different.

CHAPTER 8

Status Report on Equality

On January 25, 2002, the National Organization on Disability (NOD) released its State of the Union 2002 for Americans with Disabilities. The NOD analysis shows that Americans with disabilities remain pervasively disadvantaged in all aspects of life. Based on the findings of a late 2001 Harris Poll survey, NOD found that the terrorist attacks of September 11, 2001, had led people touched with disabilities to "reevaluate our lifestyles, and consider what we could change to better protect ourselves and our loved ones."[1]

More than ten years after the signing of the ADA, efforts to ensure equal access continue on the local, state, and national levels—evidence that much remains to be done. In communities such as Berkeley, California, disabled residents battle to make sure that personal assistance services are made available to people who need them in an emergency, and the state of Louisiana finally responded to pressure and demonstrations by ADAPT to provide more in-home services. The Florida-based Association for DisAbled Americans and the Florida Paraplegic Association have filed class action lawsuits against businesses that have failed to make their facilities and services fully accessible, as has the Disabled Rights Action Committee in Las Vegas. Many activists have fought for the right to bring their service animals into public places (such as the San Diego Zoo), and members of the National Federation of the Blind voted to opt out of a settlement with the state of Hawaii over bringing guide dogs into the state. The accessibility of over-the-road buses is still the subject of suits claiming that staff in some companies are not adequately or properly trained and do not provide assistance needed by riders with disabilities. Pennsylvania's Coalition of Citizens with Disabilities has pushed activists to file *pro se* lawsuits as a strategy to force accessibility compliance.

Each of these developments is further proof that passage of the ADA was only the beginning—that its symbolism must be reinforced through continuing activist vigilance, implementation, and enforcement. These actions also are responses to ideas that, though not new, have not been fully accepted by American society. Universal design, for example, makes buildings accessible to nondisabled persons; a ramp to a building can be used by all people, including people using baby carriages, those with walkers and wheelchairs, and elderly people. Many newspapers published comical reactions to a Federal Aviation Administration regulation (in response to the ADA) that requires accommodations for people who have allergic reactions to nuts, such as the infamous in-flight peanut. Disability policy changes remain glacial and difficult to achieve.

This chapter reviews and, in some cases, compares findings and recommendations from various reports and researchers on disability policy in the United States. Unfortunately, few studies have been conducted to measure the "success" of the ADA and other statutes, and quality of life is an elusive, difficult-to-quantify term.[2] It is possible, however, to look at several areas of American society to determine when and where policy that affects persons with disabilities has changed, in either a positive or negative sense.

There will be plausible arguments over whether persons with disabilities are better off now than they used to be. As has been the case with society in general, the overall economic gap between the "haves" and the "have nots" in the United States is growing each year. Yet there is some agreement about what measures can be used to identify and evaluate public policies that affect the population as a whole. This chapter begins with an analysis of attitudes and public opinion about disabilities to see whether long-held stereotypes have changed. The chapter then moves on to address six specific policy areas that have been identified as key indicators of progress: employment, social integration, barriers to independence, transportation, health care, and housing.

ATTITUDES AND PUBLIC OPINION

Although there is considerable anecdotal information about attitudes toward individuals with disabilities, one of the most widely cited resources is a 2000 Harris and Associates poll commissioned by NOD. The poll was conducted in May–June 2000 among a nationwide cross-section of adults with and without disabilities. Respondents were asked about ten key measures of quality of life to determine whether the past decade has seen notable improvements for people with disabilities. NOD notes that people with disabilities are not a homogenous group, and those with slight or moderate disabilities have dramatically different needs than people with somewhat or very severe disabilities. There also are substantial gaps between people with disabilities and the general population.[3] These findings are integrated into the discussion that follows.

Another widely cited survey is the 1999 Harris Poll conducted for NOD to determine the impact of the ADA. The opinion poll showed that there was support for the statute and agreement that efforts should continue to create employment opportunities, make transportation accessible, offer home care services to allow people to avoid nursing homes, and end discrimination in public places.[4]

About two-thirds of those polled in 1999 said that they had seen, heard, or read about the ADA; of that group, 87 percent favored and supported the legislation, whereas 8 percent disapproved and 5 percent did not know. When respondents were asked about specific topics, more than 80 percent felt that creating opportunities for people with disabilities would decrease welfare rolls and increase employment opportunities; only 12 percent felt that it would be very expensive and not worth the cost for employers to hire more people with disabilities. Of the total sample, 94 percent believed employers should not discriminate against any qualified job candidate with a disability, and 85 percent favored reasonable accommodations for workers with disabilities in places employing fifteen or more people. More than 90 percent favored making public transportation accessible, and 95 percent agreed that public places such as hotels, restaurants, and stores must not discriminate. With regard to nursing homes, 86 percent said that the government must offer home care services that allow more people with disabilities to live at home instead of in nursing homes.[5]

Alan Reich, president of NOD, interpreted the poll results as support for the ADA. "This survey knocks on the head any suggestion that America's commitment to ending discrimination against people with disabilities is flagging. On the contrary, we see new evidence that fundamental fairness, which is the essence of the ADA, remains a cornerstone American value."[6]

That value does not hold much promise for disabled women, however. A four-year study by the Baylor College of Medicine's Center for Research on Women with Disabilities found that society continues to have negative stereotypes about the abilities and potential of women with disabilities. "They constitute the nation's most severely oppressed minority," according to Dr. Margaret Nosek, principal investigator in the study. Women with disabilities were equally likely to experience emotional, physical, or sexual abuse as nondisabled women but did so for a longer period because of fewer options for resolving the abuse. Self-esteem was found to be much lower in women with disabilities, and respondents said they had more limited opportunities to establish romantic relationships because of their disability.[7]

Some business owners still feel that the ADA provides special treatment for persons with disabilities, and their actions indicate that they are still trying to figure how to avoid complying with the law. In 1999, for example, the Sacramento chapter of the California Restaurant Association invited members to attend a workshop on how to deal with "access blasters who target restaurants for lawsuits and attorney's fees for lack of wheelchair access to restrooms and other facilities." The notice of the meeting made clear the group's attitude toward the ADA and the concept of reasonable accommodation:

> Discover the horrors of legal blackmail and the "dirty tricks" used by enterprising plaintiff's attorneys to enhance awards and fees. Learn about the risks of non-compliance with federal and state ADA access laws and how to deal with them. Hear how to minimize potential attorney's fees you must pay to the ADA plaintiff's attorney.[8]

Although Americans favor ending discrimination and increasing inclusion, the reality of how well those values translate into policy is very different. The following sections analyze what is known about key quality-of-life indicators related to persons with disabilities. Although these indicators show that some areas are improving the lives of PWDs, there is still a large gap between policy promise and performance.

EMPLOYMENT

Increasing employment opportunities for persons with disabilities has been a key priority within disability policy for decades. One of the difficulties in formulating policy, however, has been the lack of accurate information. As with other issues, employment data suffer from several methodological problems. Along with the traditional issue of how best to define disability, researchers struggle with validity and reliability, especially in longitudinal studies.

The 2000 NOD/Harris survey found significant gaps between the employment rates of working disabled and working nondisabled people. Only 32 percent of disabled persons of working age (eighteen to sixty-four) work full or part-time, compared to 81 percent of the nondisabled population. Since 1986, the percentage of persons who say they are able to work increased from 46 percent to 56 percent; of those ages eighteen to twenty-nine, 57 percent of those with disabilities who are able to work are working. One important factor to consider is that over the past fourteen years,

the disabled population has become more severely disabled—the proportion of severely disabled people has risen from 29 percent to 43 percent—
reducing the potential number of individuals who are able to work.[9]

There is a significant gap in income levels between people who are disabled and those who are not. The 2000 survey found that 29 percent of
disabled persons had a household income of $15,000 or less, compared to
10 percent of those without disabilities. Disabled persons also were less
likely to have household incomes more than $50,000 (16 percent versus 39
percent). As with employment, younger people with disabilities had a
smaller gap (30 percent to 21 percent) in income relative to people without disabilities.[10]

Despite potential sources of error, many studies that are based on the
household Survey of Income and Program Participation (SIPP) acknowledge its usefulness as an instrument for measuring changes in the employment rate of individuals. Under SIPP definitions, individuals are considered to be employed if they worked at a job or business at any time during
the month preceding the interview month. SIPP also uses a definition of
disability that is closest to the ADA's definition.

Using data gathered from the 1991/92, 1993/94, 1994/95, and 1997 SIPPs,
one study found that the employment rate for individuals with a disability was 50.4 percent in 1994/95 and 48.1 percent in 1997. The study also
adjusted the data to differentiate between individuals with a severe disability (defined as individuals who are younger than sixty-five years old
who are covered by Medicare or are receiving Supplemental Security
Income payments—indicating a disability that prevents gainful employment) and those with a nonsevere disability. In 1994/95, 20.3 million individuals had a work disability; 8.6 million were unable to work, and 11.7
million were able to work. In the most recent sample, 1997, the number of
persons with a work disability was 16.1 million; the number unable to work
was 9.4 million, and the number able to work was 6.7 million. For those
with a severe disability, the employment rate was 34.1 percent in 1994/95
and 29.4 percent for 1997. The comparable figures for those with a nonsevere disability were 61.6 percent (1994/95) and 63.9 percent (1997).[11]

More current census data underscore the fact that unemployment rates among disabled workers are more than twice the national average. As of March 1999, the number of persons ages sixteen to seventy-four who have a condition that prevents them from working or limits the amount of work they can do was 2.1 million, with an average unemployment rate of 10.5 percent. The unemployment figures are highest among those ages sixteen to twenty-four (22.5 percent), decreasing sharply to 7.1 percent at age forty-five to fifty-four and dropping to 6.4 percent among persons with a disability in the sixty-five to sixty-nine age group.[12]

Statistics aside (and there is universal agreement that no single survey is an adequate measure of employment), what policy changes have been made to increase the employment rate among the disabled?

During the Clinton administration, two major steps were taken to facilitate new employment opportunities for persons with disabilities. In January 1999 a three-part initiative was announced that would invest more than $2 billion over a five-year period. The program included full funding of the Work Incentives Improvement Act, estimated at $1.2 billion; a $1,000 tax credit to cover work-related costs for people with disabilities, at a cost of $700 million; and $35 million for expanded access to information and communications technologies in FY 2000.[13]

The Ticket to Work program, which is voluntary, offers vocational services and employment to disabled persons ages eighteen to sixty-four who receive cash disability payments under Social Security. Individuals receive a "ticket" that allows them to work without losing their Medicare and Medicaid benefits—one of the reasons that many disabled people who are eager to work remain unemployed. The tickets can be used for training programs and job placement services through a state's employment network. Twelve states launched the program in 2002, with the rest of the nation scheduled to follow in 2003.

In a second proposal, in February 2000, the Clinton administration announced plans to create a new Office on Disability Policy, Evaluation, and Technical Assistance, with the specific charge of increasing the employment rate among people with disabilities. The action was part of DOL's proposed 2001 budget, with an initial funding level of $21 million. Under the president's proposal, the President's Committee on the Employment of People with Disabilities would be absorbed into the new agency, as recommended by committee members in their second report to the president.[14]

Despite good intentions, enforcement of the employment-related provisions of the ADA clearly is falling far short of what supporters had hoped. Litigation—regarded as the last resort in resolving Title I disputes—has failed to serve as a disincentive to some of the nation's most visible employers. On June 1, 2001, for instance, the U.S. Equal Employment Opportunity Commission (EEOC) filed its third suit against Minneapolis-based Northwest Airlines for employment policies that discriminate against disabled persons. Each of the three suits involved Northwest's failure to individually assess job applicants' ability to perform essential functions of the job; the company's hiring policies should have been revised more than ten years earlier, when the ADA was signed into law. Also in 2001, EEOC suits were filed against E.I. Dupont De Nemours and Co. and against Holiday Inn—large employers that ostensibly should be familiar with and thus compliant with the ADA.[15]

Disability rights attorneys acknowledge that filing cases against high-profile companies or organizations helps "send a message" that persons with disabilities are seriously seeking employment as well as fighting pervasive job discrimination. There is another aspect to employment, however, that remains less visible and underfunded: the vocational rehabilitation programs that were at the heart of early attempts to assist persons with disabilities in joining the workforce.

SOCIAL INTEGRATION

In 2002 NOD reported that 35 percent of people with disabilities say they are not at all involved with their communities, compared to 21 percent of persons who are not disabled. "Not surprisingly, then, those with disabilities are one and a half times as likely to feel isolated from others or left out of their community than those without disabilities."[16] Whether social integration involves participation in religious life, community activities, politics, housing, education, or housing, NOD notes that Americans with disabilities remain pervasively disadvantaged in all aspects of American life.

Voting

One of the hallmarks of a representative democracy is the free expression of opinion and the election of individuals who serve as stewards of those opinions. The primary mechanism for such expression is the voting process, although that is only one form of political participation. For disabled adults, voting is an activity that continues to be limited and often impossible. Voting rights are protected under the 1965 Voting Rights Act, which allows a disabled voter to receive assistance from a person of their choice, as well as the 1984 Voting Accessibility for the Elderly and Handicapped Act. The latter statute requires that persons with disabilities have access to auxiliary aids such as large-print ballots.

Title II of the ADA also applies to voting because it requires that all public entities make voting accessible, whether that includes modifying voting booths, providing assistance in various formats, or eliminating discriminatory practices. These issues have served as a barrier to voting for many persons with disabilities. The Federal Election Commission (FEC) issued a report in 1996 that was designed to help election officials comply with the ADA by addressing physical accessibility standards and how accommodations were to be funded. The FEC also noted, however, that election officials are not under any obligation to fund architectural changes to make a polling place accessible.[17]

Architectural impediments are only one way in which persons with disabilities face barriers to voting. In a 1997 study of voting rights for persons with cognitive and emotional disabilities, researchers found that forty-four states had specific constitutional provisions, statutes, or case law that disenfranchised various categories of disabled individuals. Some states refused to allow whole classes of people to vote (those variously termed idiots, insane, lunatics, mentally incompetent, mentally incapacitated, unsound minds, not quiet and peaceable, and under guardianship and/or conservatorship). Some of the restrictions were part of the state's original constitution, such as in Florida's 1868 document; other states added the limitations later—as in Missouri, which added language limiting voting by persons termed "idiots" or "insane" when its original 1875 constitution was amended in 1945. These types of restrictions are legal as part of a state's sovereignty and its power to conduct elections and establish voter qualifications.[18]

A second form of voter exclusion involves lack of accessible polling places or usable voting machines. This issue gained special significance in the 2000 presidential election, especially in the pivotal state of Florida. The state's Council of the Blind estimates that more than 250,000 of Florida's 9 million voters are visually impaired, and hundreds of thousands more have physical disabilities. Hundreds of Florida precincts are in churches, which are not required to comply with the ADA, and the state's infamous punch-card ballots are not user-friendly for people with disabilities.[19]

In Philadelphia, a wheelchair user who has multiple sclerosis, along with eight other plaintiffs led by NOD, sued the city demanding the constitutional right to vote. The suit, which is the first of its kind against a city, alleges that of the 1,681 polling places in Philadelphia, only 46 are accessible to wheelchair users. In addition, many of the city's voting machines are not usable by persons with limited or no vision. The goal of the suit is to get the city to commit to a date by which all polling places will be made accessible and to require the city to purchase voting machines with audio output that are accessible. A 1999 study of three upstate counties in New York found that fewer than 10 percent of polling places were fully compliant with state and federal laws.[20]

Despite these factors, persons with disabilities are becoming increasingly active in voting. In the 1996 presidential election, about half of all eligible voters cast ballots; 31 percent of PWDs voted. In the 2000 election, after significant efforts were made to increase voter registration nationally, the voting percentage among PWDs rose to 41 percent. A NOD/Harris Poll conducted by telephone just before the November 2000 election sug-

gested that Al Gore received 56 percent of the votes of persons with disabilities; George W. Bush won 38 percent, and Ralph Nader received 4 percent. If people with disabilities had voted with the same turnout as the rest
of the public (51 percent instead of 41 percent), the study predicted that
Gore would have won the popular vote by between 1 and 1.5 million votes.
Had that pattern happened uniformly across the country, Gore would have
won Florida's electoral votes and the presidency.[21]

The online advocacy group Justice For All issued an alert in March 2001
calling for congressional legislation mandating uniform accessibility of
polling places, equipment, and ballots. The group also called on Congress
to enact regulations to give blind or visually impaired voters the right to
mark their ballot in private, with the right of enforcement when those regulations are violated. Cited within the alert were statistics from the
National Voter Independence Project that in the 2000 election, 47 percent
of persons with disabilities responding to a survey had experienced some
type of difficulty attempting to vote. Thirteen percent of the respondents
had no choice but to vote outside because the polling place was not
accessible. More than 80 percent of the respondents reported that blind
and visually impaired voters did not have the ability to mark a ballot
confidentially.[22]

In an October 2001 report, the U.S. General Accounting Office used
a nationwide survey of almost 500 polling places across the United States
to determine accessibility during the 2000 elections. The study estimated
that 84 percent of polling places have some potential barriers to persons
with disabilities, especially those with mobility impairments. None of the
polling places surveyed were found to have ballots or equipment specifically adapted for blind voters, and most had barriers on the path of travel
from the parking lot to the building and the building entrance.[23]

The 1993 National Voter Registration Act (NVRA), which required
voter registration to be conducted in departments of motor vehicles, public assistance agencies, and military recruitment agencies, also contained
a provision that required agencies serving disabled persons to assist in voter
registration. A coalition of groups led by activist Jim Dickson was suc-

cessful in having the disabled services agencies included, despite bitter
fighting between Democrats and Republicans.[24] Implementation of the
NVRA has been difficult, however. A 1999 National Council on Disability
survey report on state compliance in vocational rehabilitation agencies
found such compliance "inconsistent and uncoordinated."[25] Another
study, conducted by University of Arkansas researcher Kay Schriner, found
that more than half of the private, nonprofit disability agencies surveyed
were not attempting to meet the requirements of the act, and 31 percent of
the responding agencies had not even heard of the NVRA.[26]

The overall findings indicate that most people with disabilities feel well
qualified to participate in politics and are as likely as nondisabled persons
to participate in several nonelectoral and civic activities, with the exception of voting. Participation is lowest among those who have difficulty
going outside the home—a form of isolation and confinement that is
heightened by difficulties in voting. These obstacles "marginalize many
people with disabilities, making them second-class citizens who cannot
publicly join others in exercising the right to vote, and weakening their
sense of connection to fellow citizens and mainstream society."[27]

Political Power

One of the themes throughout this book is that the hidden army of disabled and nondisabled activists that coalesced around the ADA represented
a unique coalition of individuals. Aside from the major disability-specific
groups, the coalition included gay and lesbian organizations, civil rights
groups, parents of disabled children, members of Congress, housing and
health care advocates, labor leaders, and women's groups (see chapter 4).

With the signing of the ADA, however, the coalition appears to have
disintegrated as the stakeholders went back to fighting the same battles the
statute was supposed to end. In recent years activism has focused on
expanding health care, enforcing the provisions of the ADA, and implementing court decisions and federal regulations. Some attempts have been
made to mobilize persons with disabilities by urging them to participate

in the political process as individuals. Prior to the 2000 election, Senator Tom Harkin and activist Justin Dart sent a message to the disability community warning that Republican leaders sought to repeal the ADA and might block legislation to guarantee people with disabilities access to health care. Harkin urged voters to support Democrats "who will build on and not destroy the progress we've made." Dart echoed, "Get involved in this election as if your lives depended upon it. They do."[28]

On a few occasions, disability groups have come together to support legislation (such as ADAPT's demonstrations on behalf of the Medicaid Community Attendant Services and Supports Act of 1999) or to protest when they believe there is discrimination against persons with disabilities. In 2001 activists sent letters and held demonstrations urging the U.S. Supreme Court to stay the scheduled execution of John Paul Penry, who had scored at the mentally retarded level in intelligence tests. The court ruled, in a 6–3 decision, that Penry could not be executed on charges of murder and rape because of the way jurors had been instructed at the sentencing phase of his trial. Although the Court did not agree with protestors who argued that the death penalty for people with mental retardation constituted cruel and unusual punishment prohibited by the Eighth Amendment to the Constitution, it reversed that view in 2002.

Most organizations still use traditional methods to bring attention to their issues, such as letter-writing campaigns and one-on-one lobbying of members of Congress. ADAPT protestors continue their tactic of disrupting meetings to put pressure on transportation firms to make buses and other forms of transit fully accessible. They remain the one major group that is most likely to participate in demonstrations for disability rights—as well as the most visible.

Political power among advocacy and service organizations has been concentrated in Washington, D.C., where such groups have greatest access to the federal government and the programs it provides. Many of the mainstream groups have offices in the Washington area that provide them geographic proximity to Congress and federal agencies (see Box 8.1). This is especially true of legal advocacy groups such as the Disability Rights

BOX 8.1

National Disability Organizations with Offices in the Washington, D.C., Area

Alexander Graham Bell Association for the Deaf

American Association of People with Disabilities

American Association of the Deaf-Blind

American Association on Mental Retardation

American Bar Association Commission on Mental and Physical Disability Law

American Council of the Blind

American Diabetes Foundation

Autism Society of America

Bazelon Center for Mental Health Law

Cochlear Implant Association

Consortium for Citizens with Disabilities

Council for Exceptional Children

Epilepsy Foundation

International Dyslexia Association

Lupus Foundation of America

Mental Disability Rights International

National Association for the Mentally Ill

National Association of the Deaf

National Association of Protection and Advocacy Systems

National Council on Independent Living

National Federation of the Blind

National Mental Health Association

National Organization on Disability

National Osteoporosis Foundation

National Parent Network on Disability

National Spinal Cord Injury Association

Paralyzed Veterans of America

Self Help for Hard of Hearing People

Spina Bifida Association of America

TASH

United Cerebral Palsy Association (UCP National)

Very Special Arts

Education and Defense Fund (DREDF), which maintains offices in Berkeley and Washington. The California office helps in the acquisition and screening of potential claims, aided by legal staff in both cities.

The difference between Washington-based groups and those outside the Beltway is significant. Those located close to the Capitol tend to be the ones with a national membership and, more important, a primary mission of advocacy. Their proximity allows them to monitor legislation and regulations and to have regular contact with members of Congress and agency leaders. In contrast, most of the other groups (many of which are identified in Appendix C) are more likely to take on the role of direct client service providers. They may serve a regional client base or be a chapter of another, larger group. They cannot afford the cost of a second office to lobby in Washington and instead may form coalitions with the groups that do have that ability. Most offer support and referral to anyone who seeks assistance, rarely requiring the formalities of membership. Some organizations are not "groups" in the formal sense but online organizations that do not have offices, meetings, boards of directors, or officers.

The availability of government grants, private philanthropic funding, and charitable organization tax benefits has enabled several groups to present themselves as having a national reputation while they are being run out of an individual's home. Some have set themselves up as "umbrella organizations" representing a long list of other groups, even though they have little influence or political impact. Others appear to be more active in promoting merchandise or an affinity credit card than in providing services, and some seem to be simply a way of providing a salary to a single person. The duplication and overlap of interests, often with names that are confusingly similar, make it difficult to determine which ones actually have power and which do not. An "association" or "institute" in fact may be little more than an Internet presence.

With minor exceptions, the potential power of the disability rights movement remains politically fragmented, as the preceding chapters have shown. Although the movement remains focused on the rights of persons with disabilities, it still is sometimes unable to stray from the needs of indi-

vidual factions, usually based on a specific type of disability. The antago-
nism of groups fighting for scarce resources manifests itself in intolerance
toward the movement's own members. In an e-mail message sent to a
widely distributed list, one California leader notes:

> It is curious and not a little disturbing how little regard some of us exhibit for
> each other when we disagree. People are demonized and slandered. . . . And
> the irony is that we generally want the same things. It is so sad to see this hap-
> pening. We need to hold together, support each other, as individuals as well
> as a community, because the real "enemies" are those who would deny us
> individuality and independence. . . . There must be another way to do this.[29]

Barriers to Independence

People with disabilities face many barriers in their lives—some of them
physical, such as racks of clothing placed too closely together in a department store that hinder a person using a wheelchair. Other barriers limit
mobility, such as cracked sidewalks without curb cuts or the lack of public transit. Outmoded attitudes and the refusal to "see" invisible disabilities keep others from socializing or joining community life. Some of these
barriers involve gaining accessibility to neighborhood restaurants; others
involve high-profile public places and services. Lawsuits and complaints
have been filed against American MultiCinema, one of the nation's largest
chains of movie theaters; Chevron gas stations; New York's Radio City
Music Hall; Ames department stores; and the health maintenance organization Kaiser Permanente. Many of the lawsuits end with settlement
agreements rather than going to trial.

Some parts of the country seem to be taking the ADA more seriously
than others, making a real attempt to make cities accessible. *New Mobility*
magazine researched the best places to live for people using wheelchairs; it
used a variety of variables to determine which ones were "disability-
friendly" (see Box 8.2). The publication contacted Centers for Independent
Living and local residents, looking not only for a lack of physical or archi-

BOX 8.2

Ten Disability-Friendly Cities

1. Denver, Colorado
2. Berkeley, California
3. Seattle, Washington
4. Sioux Falls, South Dakota
5. Raleigh, North Carolina
6. San Jose, California
7. Salt Lake City, Utah
8. Rochester, Minnesota
9. Madison, Wisconsin
10. Albuquerque, New Mexico

Almost Made the List: Topeka, Kansas; Gainesville, Sarasota, and St. Petersburg, Florida; Minneapolis and St. Paul, Minnesota; Ithaca, New York; Philadelphia, Pennsylvania

Source: Cindy McCoy, "10 Disability-Friendly Cities," *New Mobility* (December 1997), 19–25.

tectural barriers but also for whether personal assistance and transportation services, support and advocacy programs, and recreational and cultural opportunities were available.

The magazine gave its highest ranking to Denver, noting the city's multitude of services and conveniences and its exceptionally strong advocacy record. Denver also is home to ADAPT, activist residents of independent living centers, and the disability support organization Atlantis Community.

Two issues are at the heart of attempts to break down barriers by opening up buildings and communication: universal design and accessible technology. These approaches represent nonstatutory advances that are changing life not only for people with disabilities but for all citizens.

Universal Design

The late architect Ron Mace developed the term *universal design* in the 1970s as a way of encouraging builders, designers, and architects to design spaces or products that are usable by everyone, regardless of their ability or disability level. The concept is intended not only to make products or buildings compliant with the ADA but also to increase the potential base of users. Mace, who was a wheelchair user, sought to redesign his own world in 1974 by helping to create the country's first building code with a section on handicapped access.[30]

Universal design grew out of the barrier-free environment movement that began in the mid-1950s. Disabled veterans and others with disabilities sought ways of becoming reintegrated into society rather than being hospitalized or placed in nursing homes. They recognized that architectural barriers reduced their opportunities for employment and education and called on Congress and the president to take steps to bring the barriers down. At about the same time, a new discipline—rehabilitation engineering—developed to create new assistive devices and prosthetics for people with disabilities, with much of the funding provided by the Veterans' Administration. The 1961 accessibility standards created by the American National Standards Institute (ANSI) were a first step in this direction, although it would take a second round of legislation at the state and local levels to provide enforcement. By 1966 thirty states had done so; by 1973 forty-nine states had adopted accessibility legislation. Unfortunately, the result was a patchwork of different standards, administrative bodies, and laws that in reality provided no standard at all. It was not until 1984 that ANSI specifications became part of the Uniform Federal Accessibility Standard, providing a way of incorporating the various state statutes in a national standard.[31] Later, universal design would incorporate the issue of multiple chemical sensitivity and the need to make all environments more universally usable, reducing the use of toxic building materials, solvents, and other pollutants.

Often features that are a part of universal design can be incorporated into a building's initial planning rather than as modifications or retrofitting. For instance, when the city of San Francisco built its new public library, architects included a sweeping interior ramp that leads from the main entryway into the atrium. Although the ramp might be regarded as a way of creating wheelchair access for patrons, even a short visit shows that the ramp is more likely to be used by persons with strollers, people using canes or walkers, individuals who walk slowly, or even able-bodied persons who are avoiding the crowded stairs. There is no signage indicating that the ramp's use is only for persons with disabilities, and the public clearly does not interpret it that way. The ramp's design helps it blend into the overall architecture of the building entryway, rather than making it seem as if it had been added as a modification or afterthought.

The principle shows up in product design as well: A telephone whose ringer can be adjusted manually allows a mother to turn the sound down so the ring does not wake her sleeping infant. It also gives a person who is hearing impaired the ability to raise the volume to the highest level. Neither requires a specially built telephone or adaptive equipment to meet their needs. The same is true for playground equipment that meets the requirements of the ADA while allowing smaller children to climb and swing. The School of Design at North Carolina State University, which was founded by Mace, opened in 1989; it serves as a universal design research center so that students and faculty can put the concept into practice. Its Design Advisory Network also provides the expertise of more than 1,000 people with disabilities who can provide valuable feedback on modifications and features to determine whether they are truly accessible.

Universal design is not universally accepted, however. At the First International Conference on Universal Design, held at Hofstra University in New York in June 1998, many of the participants from universities shared their experiences of being told that the concept was too narrow a specialty or that they had found administrative resistance to adding courses on universal design to the curriculum. To counter that obstacle, the terms "design for aging," "UD," or "design for all people" often are used instead. Another measure of the lack of full acceptance of the concept is that the number of academic institutions that participated in the Universal Design

Education Project dropped from more than twenty schools to just nine in a few short years.[32]

Mace, who died in 1998, was honored with the Distinguished Service Award of the President of the United States by President George Bush in 1992; he also was a fellow of the American Institute of Architects and a research professor at North Carolina State University. His legacy of universal design, despite its potential and promise, has not helped to improve the lives of all people, as he had hoped. Yet for persons with disabilities who can now open a can of soup, for older persons who can now gain access to the large-print section of their local library, or for a person without a disability who finds the perfect home, universal design is a measure of progress.

Assistive Technology and Electronic Accessibility

One of the areas in which there has been great progress in equalizing the lives of persons with disabilities is in technology and its subsector, assistive technology. Since 1973 companies doing business with the federal government have been required to provide accommodations. Now driven by the reasonable accommodation provisions of Title I of the ADA, employers are finding that with a minimal investment, they can hire from a large pool of talented workers by making the workplace accessible.

Assistive technology for persons with disabilities often has been the precursor for devices that later benefit society as a whole. For example, the typewriter was invented to enable blind people to write for sighted readers without translation from Braille. Today's ubiquitous computer modem started out as an "acoustic coupler" developed in the early 1960s by deaf physicist Robert H. Weitbrecht. The device was intended to help deaf people send messages over standard telephone lines by using a teletypewriter, or TTY.[33]

Since that time, a wide range of tools have enabled PWDs to gain independence in ways never thought of a decade ago. The Kurzweil Reading Edge optical scanner allows blind users to convert written words to spoken text; Voice Information Associates, a market research company, estimates that the market for speech-to-text products will exceed $4.3 billion by the end of 2001. In Sherman Oaks, California, the General Cinema Theatre in 1997 became the first conventional movie theater to install two new technologies for moviegoers. The Rear Window Captioning System allows deaf and hearing-impaired patrons to view text on a portable acrylic screen, allowing them to sit anywhere in the theater. DVS Theatrical provides narration through a listening system, enabling blind or visually impaired customers to hear descriptions on headsets without disturbing others in the theater.[34] In June 1999 Wells Fargo Bank and the California Council of the Blind announced that Wells Fargo would pilot the first talking automatic teller machines (ATMs). The devices instruct users on how to deposit money, withdraw cash, transfer funds, and buy stamps, enabling vision-impaired customers to have access to information they could not read on a regular ATM screen.[35] Each of these developments has opened everyday experiences to millions of people who previously had to rely on others for assistance or were left out of the communication loop entirely.

An emerging technology issue is the use and accessibility of the Internet. Originally the Internet was designed to be used in text-only format. As the technology expanded, web pages were created with visual and sound prompts, such as graphic images and background music related to the site. Although this new form of communication opened the world for many users who are disabled, it created additional barriers for others with vision or hearing impairments.

Access to the Internet is included under the federal regulations that require covered entities to furnish appropriate auxiliary aids and services where necessary as a way of ensuring effective communication with individuals with disabilities. These methods of communication may include the use of materials in Braille or large print, captioning, audiotaped books and text, and other methods to make media accessible. Although the emphasis has been on people with visual impairments, those who are deaf or hearing impaired lack accessibility to audio messages and music, which are becoming more common.

Public and private entities are covered, so government agencies, businesses, and services that are available to the public must make Internet communication (such as websites) fully accessible. As web commerce has developed, there is a parallel need for accessibility of sites whose primary source of business is the online customer. Similarly, municipal governments that proudly hail the development of a city services website, complete with video coverage of city council meetings and hearings, must realize that not all citizens can see or hear what is going on. Even institutions of higher education are beginning to realize the need to make distance learning (often via the Internet or interactive television) or library resources available to all students, including those who are disabled.

The city of San Jose, California, was among the first to embrace the ADA and develop a standard for accessibility to its web pages. In June 1996 the city established seven minimum requirements to ensure web accessibility; those standards were cited as part of a best practices model by the League of California Cities. Some other cities have followed San Jose's lead, but many local and state government agencies have not.

On the federal level, however, the Rehabilitation Act Amendments of 1998 required all federal agencies to make their websites, information technology, and telecommunications equipment accessible by June 21, 2001. The amendments had a loophole, however, in that they required that agencies were to solidify their plans for becoming technologically accessible by the deadline but did not require that accessibility be fully implemented. Journalist John Williams reported that several private companies were rushing to meet the deadline because the law also covers vendors who sell their products to the federal government. Despite reassurances from vendors and the Information Technology Association of America, however, Williams criticizes the lack of planning, commenting, "They knew Section 508 regulations were coming, yet only a small handful have taken the initiative to promote accessibility."[36]

San Jose's former ADA coordinator, Cynthia Waddell, terms the problems encountered by persons with disabilities a "digital divide." She uses the term to describe the lack of accessible web design and its effect on those persons' ability to have access to employment and commerce. "There is an affirmative duty to develop a comprehensive policy involving input from the community of people with disabilities. New technology must either improve accessibility or ensure compatibility with existing design functions."[37]

Disabled citizens and customers report their inability to access important government information or conduct business online. Yet the need is there even for people who do not use a computer or the Internet. They have difficulty using household appliances with touch-screen or flat-screen displays, such as microwaves and ovens. This is one of the last frontiers for barrier removal, but it also is crucial for persons with disabilities who want to become fully integrated into society. As Waddell notes, "Overcoming the digital divide for people with disabilities requires a 'free and fair flow of information' safeguarded by civil rights. Civil rights principles should guide policymakers in the application of technology in the emerging digital economy. Although information technology changes, civil rights principles do not."[38]

Advanced technology is worth little, however, if it is not made available to persons who need to use it. Traditionally, public libraries have served as technology havens, with free access to scanners, the Internet, assistive listening devices, electronic print enlargers, and synthetic speech and screen-reading software. A 1998 American Library Association (ALA) study found, however, that of the 15,718 libraries surveyed, only 2.9 percent had special software or hardware for use by persons with disabilities at all library workstations, and 83.6 percent had no special access workstations at all.[39] Although some metropolitan libraries have installed the most innovative technologies and made their facilities user-friendly (for example, in San Francisco, Phoenix, and San Diego), many others have made no provisions for disabled persons. The ALA is one of the leading organizations attempting to improve services for patrons with disabilities; it has developed a Learning Disabilities Initiative to increase libraries' capacities in this area.

TRANSPORTATION

Prior to passage of the ADA, disabled persons routinely were denied the ability to use public transit systems and other forms of transportation. Stephanie Thomas, ADAPT organizer, notes that transportation, both symbolically and in reality, is the key to linking with others. "Mobility, the ability to get out, to get around and connect with other people, is fundamental to being a part of a larger community."[40] Disability activists have believed that focusing on transportation also was part of their efforts to gain dignity and respect by making their own decisions about getting around. Attorney Timothy Cook found that few of the court cases brought by disability groups to obtain accessible buses were successful prior to the ADA, primarily because the judiciary held that the 1973 Rehabilitation Act did not require integrated services.[41]

Many activists acknowledge that segregated transit modes (especially those marked as "handicapped only" or "Reserved for Handicapped") are no different from buses that segregated persons of color from whites. In a 1950 U.S. Supreme Court case, the justices ruled that having one table in a railroad dining car designated for Negroes was unreasonably prejudicial and served only to call attention to discriminatory treatment.[42] To some activists in the disability community, "special" transportation is much the same.

During the ADA hearings, however, Congress made clear its intent to eliminate "separate but equal" practices. Senator Edward Kennedy called for an end to "this American apartheid. [The ADA] will roll back the unthinking and unacceptable practices by which disabled Americans today are segregated, excluded, and fenced off from fair participation in our society by mindless biased attitudes and senseless physical barriers."[43]

When consumers with disabilities were asked in the 2000 NOD/Harris survey whether inadequate transportation is considered a problem, 30 percent of those responding answered yes, as opposed to only 10 percent of those who do not have disabilities. The problem is particularly acute among those persons with very severe or somewhat severe disabilities (35 percent thought transportation was a problem). The lack of adequate transportation for any group reduces the opportunity to get to work or school or to meet with friends and socialize. Among people with disabilities, this problem leads to increasing social isolation and unemployment.[44]

How much real progress has there been? In 2002 NOD reported that 30 percent of persons with disabilities often have insufficient access to transportation—three times the rate of nondisabled persons. "This creates a Catch-22 situation: How can one have a job if one cannot get to it? How can one afford transportation if one does not have a job?"[45]

With regard to air travel, passengers with disabilities not only face the usual problems of delays and lost baggage; they also face accessibility problems. Although Congress enacted the Air Carrier Access Act in 1986, airlines sometimes have refused to allow disabled passengers to board flights, required a nondisabled person to accompany them, or charged higher fees. When a disabled person does fly, the passenger often has difficulty getting onto the aircraft because the only way to board is by using a staircase leading to a narrow aisle. Disabled passengers may be treated discourteously by airline staff who have little or no training in dealing with the needs of persons with disabilities. Often the airports themselves are still inaccessible, with restrooms that cannot accommodate a wheelchair, lack of signage or audible signals, or too few handicapped parking areas. About 100 ADAPT protestors targeted Kansas City International Airport in February 2001 seeking equal access within the airport as well as accessible transit and shuttle buses.

Prior to 1998, these problems often were not fully documented because passengers with disabilities did not file formal complaints. The U.S. Department of Transportation (DOT) did not separate disability-related consumer complaints against U.S. airlines until 1998, so the number and magnitude of reported cases with boarding, baggage, or other problems is very sketchy. DOT's Office of Consumer Affairs has now begun to collect this information, however, and it reports a 63 percent increase in complaints from 1998 to 1999. Still, much information on what progress has been made remains to be reported or researched.

During the Clinton administration, Secretary of Transportation Rodney E. Slater announced a policy statement in support of a fully accessible transportation system, saying the goal "is not only essential but attainable."[46] The new policies, released on the tenth anniversary of the signing of the ADA, included creation of an accessibility task force, an initiative on pedestrian access to comply with the ADA, a broad set of new rules for modification of vehicles to meet the needs of persons with disabilities, and funding for training and capital costs to make over-the-road buses wheelchair accessible.

Complaints to the U.S. Department of Justice (DOJ) and litigation seem to have become the most effective strategies used by disability rights groups to gain access to transportation. For example, Disability Rights Advocates sued on behalf of eight disabled riders to force San Francisco's Bay Area Rapid Transit system (BART) to comply with the ADA. The focus of the suit was not just accessibility (BART previously had agreed to spend $55.4 million on accessibility) but maintenance of the system's elevators, lowering the height of fare machines and telephones, and cleaning its trains more frequently. The settlement agreement included about $650,000 in free fares for the estimated 1,500 BART riders who are disabled and $100,000 for Bay-area independent living centers.

In one of the most sweeping settlements, Greyhound Bus Lines agreed to resolve complaints filed with DOJ by passengers with disabilities. In the September 24, 1999, agreement, the company said it would phase in accessible bus service, provide training to all employees in assisting any person with a disability, continue systematically removing barriers to access in Greyhound facilities, and inform individuals with disabilities of their rights. Greyhound previously had been subject to 1998 DOT regulations that all newly purchased or leased buses be lift-equipped by October 2000. The agreement gave the company an additional year to comply but required that meaningful access be provided in the interim. This requirement included a provision that Greyhound would make reasonable efforts to provide accessible bus service in its service area with forty-eight hours' notice. The fourteen complainants—who reported verbal harassment, experienced boarding difficulties, or were refused passage—received damage awards of $500 to $4,000.[47] Such high-profile cases and agreements move implementation forward, but the actions often take years to resolve, limiting one of the most important resources of persons with disabilities—the ability to travel freely.

HEALTH CARE

Health care has been at the top of the policy agenda for the past several years, and it is of special interest to persons with disabilities. NOD surveys show that health care is less accessible to people with disabilities, who often need it most, often because of limited employment and reduced discretionary income, along with transportation barriers. An estimated 28 percent of PWDs delay getting needed health care because they cannot afford it, compared to 12 percent of the general population.[48] There has been little research into the subject of whether persons with disabilities are getting "better" services in the post-ADA decade or whether those services are more accessible regardless of the type of disability. There is evidence that the issue of mental retardation is receiving more attention, but health care is not. A February 2002 report by the U.S. Surgeon General found that the U.S. health care system has "failed to respond to changes in the lives of people with mental retardation"; the report offered a series of recommendations from a national conference.[49]

Two areas in which health care policy is most crucial are the use of personal attendant services and access to health care facilities.

Personal Attendant Services

One of the most enduring issues in disability policy is the need for alternatives to nursing homes and other institutions for individuals who need long-term services. Historically, there has been an institutional bias because every state that receives Medicaid funding from the federal government must provide nursing home services, whereas community-based services are optional. TASH (formerly the Association for Persons with Severe Handicaps) estimates that more than 80 percent of Medicaid dollars, or about $41 billion, supports institutional care, whereas only 20 percent is spent on programs within the community, even though studies show the latter to be less expensive.[50]

An attempt to provide services in the most integrated setting, the Medicaid Community Attendant Services Act (MiCASA), was introduced into Congress by former Speaker of the House Newt Gingrich (R-GA) in 1997. Although the bill had bipartisan support, it died when the legislative session ended. In 1999 a revised (and slightly renamed) bill, the Medicaid Community Attendant Services and Supports Act (MiCASSA), was introduced by Senators Tom Harkin (D-IA) and Arlen Specter (R-PA) with the input of many organizations with a stake in long-term services and supports. The main feature of the bill was that it would funnel funds directly to individuals rather than to service providers or institutions. This provision would allow consumers to choose what kinds of care they required, including the use of unlicensed personal attendants. States would not be required to spend more money under this plan than they did prior to its passage; the difference lies in the types of programs that would be funded.

ADAPT members have made passage of MiCASSA one of their main goals, demonstrating on the bill's behalf in Washington, D.C. The revised bill had less support than the 1997 measure, in part because it was introduced late in the congressional session and in part because of concerns about its costs.[51] In May 2002, thousands of activists participated in a "phone-in" in Washington in support of MiCASSA, asking President Bush to make the program part of his New Freedom initiative.

MiCASSA has been opposed, not unexpectedly, by lobbyists for the nursing home industry, as well as by nursing organizations. The latter group is opposed to any measure that would delegate certain types of medical procedures to non-nursing staff. Delegation is restricted by Nurse Practice Acts in effect in all fifty states. DREDF and other advocacy groups are seeking to end these statutes, which protect nursing jobs and, some say, make caring for disabled persons more expensive than if a personal atten-

dant were to perform the same function. Nurses respond that the laws protect patients by requiring professional standards and regulating the quality of care.

Kansas amended its Nurse Practice Act in 1989 so that "nursing-related
tasks" can be performed by personal attendants. The amendment was part
of a shift toward consumer-controlled services; it saved the state an estimated $52 million in Medicaid costs in 1998. Nebraska also has amended
its statute to allow a competent individual to direct a designated caregiver
to provide health maintenance activities—defined as things that the individual would perform if he or she were physically able. As one critic of the
Nurse Practice Acts notes, "[the acts show a] lack of consideration for the
impact these laws have on people" and "an unintended consequence [that]
was never a part of the discussion."[52]

As a result, personal attendant services vary considerably from state to
state and region to region. In communities where activists within the disability community have been especially vigilant—such as Berkeley,
California—the issue has been supported by residents and the local city
council. In other areas, the absence of a sufficient pool of well-trained
personal assistants can reduce social integration and lead to medical
emergencies.

Health Care Facilities

The health care issue exploded in 1999 when the U.S. Supreme Court (in
the *Olmstead* decision described in greater detail in chapter 7) required
states to offer services "in the most integrated setting." As a result, state
legislatures began the long process of amending laws and increasing funding for community-based services. In Texas, the legislature voted to use the
"money follows the individual" policy, which allows a person to leave a
nursing home, with the same amount of money spent there to be used for
community/personal services. In Wisconsin, nursing home operators
claimed that legislators were stealing from them when the state voted to
provide $50 million for community-based services for seniors and people

with developmental disabilities.[53] Still, there are limitations. A Missouri official wrote disability advocates that "the state's obligation to provide community-based services is not boundless. No state is required under this [*Olmstead*] ruling to dismantle its current institutional system to fund clients who want community placement."[54]

Still unresolved, however, is accessibility of health care facilities—an issue that the ADA was supposed to have resolved. As Boston University School of Law researcher Lawrence O. Gostin notes, the ADA made clear that the professional office of a health care provider, a hospital, or other service provider was included under the public accommodations portion of the statute. The law, Gostin writes, does not guarantee access to health care: it merely requires that refusal to provide equal access cannot be based on a person's disability. The ADA also does not distinguish between health care decisions that are made on a purely financial basis (such as not treating a patient who does not have the ability to pay) and subtle forms of discrimination (such as referring a patient with a disability to another physician or provider). "The ADA, then, in only a limited sense tears down barriers to access to health services. . . . It remains uncertain as to what extent the act will help to ensure access to health care for those who arguably need it most."[55]

One wheelchair user writes of her experiences in a hospital emergency room, which are not atypical. An emergency room nurse who had not carefully read the admissions intake forms asked the woman—who was paraplegic—if she could stand and pivot; an orderly asked if she needed help getting into bed. ("Unless the bed can be lowered to wheelchair height, then yes I will need help," she responded.) When she was sent to the x-ray department, there was no accessible table for the procedure. One nurse was unfamiliar with the catheterization procedure used to obtain a urine specimen. The patient experienced similar problems at an optometrist's office, her personal physician's office, and while getting a mammogram. None of the facilities had accessible tables; they relied on staff to lift her.[56] Although patients without disabilities might receive similar treatment (long waits to see a physician, confusion over medical forms, impersonal treatment), for those who do need well-trained staff in a hospital setting, the emergency room can become a nightmare.

The issue is not related to technology; manufacturers already have made accessible examination tables and chairs (such as those used in a dentist's office, which can be raised and lowered), and many modifications are simple and inexpensive. Moving tables and chairs to provide a clear path of travel, adding a small ramp to a restroom, and training staff in the needs of persons with disabilities would seem to be easily implemented.

HOUSING

Most of the housing stock in the United States was not originally designed or built with the needs of persons with disabilities in mind. Prior to passage of the ADA, the 1990 National Health Interview Survey found that only 2.9 percent of Americans lived in housing with accessible features such as ramps, raised-level toilets, or extra-wide doors.[57]

Some of the policies that limited housing for persons with disabilities were eliminated or have been litigated since passage of the 1968 Fair Housing Act (FHA) and the Fair Housing Amendments Act of 1988 (FHAA). The 1988 amendments, for example, prohibited apartment owners from refusing to rent to a person with a disability. New multi-unit housing (four or more units constructed after March 13, 1991) were required to include certain accessibility features to make them adaptable. Further protections were offered by Section 504 of the Rehabilitation Act Amendments of 1973. The statutes cover various types of housing, and although they are not directed specifically at the disability community they have had an impact in opening neighborhoods and residences that previously excluded them. Most of the changes have applied to multi-family housing, however, rather than single-family residences.

Two titles of the 1990 ADA further strengthened protections against housing discrimination faced by disabled people. Title II, which covers local and state governments and provision of public services, applies to any housing that is planned, developed, managed, leased, or owned by these government entities. Title III, which is applicable to places of public accommodation, covers the entities or individuals who own, lease, or operate the accommodation—which includes places of lodging and social service center establishments. Although the first category is self-explanatory, the second also is important because it has been interpreted to include facilities such as homeless shelters, nursing homes, and any other place where a person may reside for varying lengths of time.

Housing policies developed as a result of these statutes have been inconsistent and difficult to enforce. Most conflicts over regulations promulgated by DOJ to implement the housing provisions of the ADA, for example, have been resolved on a case-by-case basis. Much of this conflict is related to the intricacy of zoning and land-use laws adopted by different jurisdictions, as well as additional requirements that are applicable to facilities that receive financial assistance from the federal government. Even the Fair Housing Act Amendments do not force an owner of a covered property to make an apartment or room accessible; instead, the legislation places the financial burden on the occupant.

More important, perhaps, statutes and regulations can do nothing to increase the *amount* of accessible housing stock that is available. In communities dominated by tract homes and with few multifamily housing options, developers seldom build houses with the needs of a person with a disability, or even an elderly person, as a guide. Conversions during new construction can be inexpensive and simple; once a home is built, the cost and feasibility to create an accessible shower, for instance, soar. In a high-rise tower, modifying a small elevator to meet the space needs of an individual in a battery-powered scooter may be prohibitive.

The *State of the Union 2002* report by NOD did not even mention the issue of housing, and it is difficult to determine whether there is a nationwide trend toward making housing more accessible. Anecdotal information suggests that persons with disabilities in cities such as San Francisco, Berkeley, and San Jose often are placed on waiting lists for accessible houses or apartments. Availability is complicated by the fact that single-family homes in those three cities are among the most expensive in the country.

Visitability—building single-family homes where persons with disabilities could not only live but visit their friends—is one of the more politicized housing-related issues. The National Association of Homebuilders has opposed regulations that require builders to include access features in new construction. Pioneering cities and localities such as Atlanta; Austin, Texas; Naperville, Illinois; Urbana, Illinois; and Pima County, Arizona, have passed visitability ordinances for newly constructed single-family homes that require wider doors and passageways, at least one no-step entrance, strategically placed light switches, and, when needed, reinforced bathroom walls that allow installation of grab bars. The concept, developed by the activist group Concrete Changes, increases building costs by an average of $265 per home. Yet those homes are usable not just by people with disabilities but by anyone with an aging family member or a child with a disability.[58] There is room for continuing comprehensive study in this area.

OVERALL ANALYSIS

Given the limitations of existing research, one can easily dismiss the impact of the ADA and other disability policies by arguing that the glass is half-full or half-empty. For activists who demand and expect immediate inclusion and economic and social parity, the glass is half-empty, and the tap is not even running under the administration of President George W. Bush. For those who are veterans of disability rights activism, the glass is half-full—an improvement over the glass that once was virtually empty.

One measure of the effects of policy change can be seen in the National Council on Disability's (NCD) third report to President Bill Clinton, *Promises to Keep: A Decade of Federal Enforcement of the Americans with Disabilities Act.* The study—part of a series that began in 1999—is an independent analysis of federal enforcement of the ADA from 1990 to 1999. It focuses on the activities of five major federal departments and agencies: DOJ, EEOC, DOT, the Federal Communications Commission, and the Architectural and Transportation Barriers Compliance Board.[59]

In the report's generally optimistic executive summary, the NCD notes that the ADA "has begun to transform the social fabric of our nation. It has brought the principle of disability rights into the mainstream of public policy. The law, coupled with the disability rights movement that produced a climate in which such legislation could be enacted, has fundamentally affected the way Americans perceive disability."[60] The document also states, however, that federal agencies charged with enforcement and policy development under the ADA have been "overly cautious, reactive, and lacking any coherent and unifying national strategy." The report also criticizes the agencies for their failure to take a leadership role in clarifying emergent issues, much of which is related to chronic underfunding and understaffing. The net effect "has been to allow the destructive effects of discrimination to continue without sufficient challenge in some quarters." The ADA enforcement agencies are characterized as "agonizingly slow" in enforcing the law and resolving complaints.[61]

The NCD report mirrors observations and public opinion surveys conducted since the passage of the ADA. More than ten years after the statute was signed, there is agreement that although the quality of life for disabled Americans has improved somewhat, the law itself has not been enough to change attitudes, significantly increase employment opportunities, end discrimination, remove barriers, or guarantee full inclusion in American society. Political scientist Stephen L. Percy notes that the magnitude of compliance responsibility extends to thousands of governing units and hundreds of thousands of business enterprises. "Despite the importance of the ADA as civil rights legislation, Congress has had no hearings on the law since its enactment, and practically no federal funds have been allocated for research on the effectiveness of ADA implementation."[62]

Berkeley researcher Frederick Collignon developed another way of measuring "success." After reviewing indicators such as benefit/cost ratios, client satisfaction, and compliance, Collignon argues that the highest-priority indicator of individual welfare should be employment, work, and income. "Higher levels of income are a means to greater consumption, better health care and other services, and a higher standard and quality of life," he notes, along with reducing dependency and the cost of social transfer payments. Collignon believes that total earnings, the percentage of persons with disabilities reporting some paid employment, the percentage of employed persons who earn at least the minimum wage, and the percentage of those whose income falls below the poverty level are the key indicators. He also recognizes, however, the need to define and measure indicators such as equal opportunity, fuller participation, and independent living. Other indicators, such as the number of persons with health insurance coverage or the percentage completing a high school education, are difficult to measure because they were not specifically part of the ADA's intent.[63]

One other measure is how persons with disabilities feel about their lives since passage of the ADA. The 2000 NOD/Harris survey found that 63 percent of all persons with disabilities, and 73 percent of persons with slight disabilities, believe that life has improved for the disabled population over the past decade. The study concludes that although a strong economy and a substantial growth in technology are responsible to some degree, "It is reasonable to attribute at least some of this progress to the implementation of the Americans with Disabilities Act of 1990."[64]

Other observers believe that success has been minimal, based on the levels of public ignorance, myths, and stereotypes that have continued to make persons with disabilities second-class citizens. Some policy changes involve political partisanship—especially those involving a conservative president and an equally conservative Supreme Court. Disability rights activism also mirrors the issue-attention cycle proposed by Anthony Downs—a process that is continuous but not predictable. Downs' cycle ebbs and flows, from initial excitement as a problem is first identified to a period of quiet inaction and disinterest.[65]

Although many activists within the disability community believe that civil rights and an end to discrimination are (or at least should be) at the top of the policy agenda, other issues and problems regularly displace those concerns. The economy, for example, is almost always among the problems mentioned as "most important" by Americans in public opinion polls. Guaranteeing equality for persons with disabilities does not even make the "top ten" list.

One could argue that passage of the ADA and other changes in disability policy reflect a unique combination of factors at a particular point in time that brought civil rights issues to the forefront. At just the right moment, activists joined legislators, people with physical disabilities joined with those who were vision- or hearing-impaired, and the policy window opened just long enough for the ADA to gain sufficient votes for passage. The conclusion of this book is that such a coalition of forces is unlikely to have the same opportunity again. Instead, continued litigation, even in the face of a more conservative judiciary, appears to be the most effective and timely way of ensuring that the promise of the ADA will be fulfilled.

Epilogue

In a May 2002 speech at Georgetown University Law School, U.S. Supreme Court Justice Sandra Day O'Connor told a lawyer's conference that the Court's recent attention to disability rights cases was the result of holes in the Americans with Disabilities Act. "It's an example of what happens when . . . the sponsors are so eager to get something passed that what passes hasn't been as carefully written as what a group of law professors might put together," O'Connor said. Saying that the 2001–2002 term would probably be remembered as the "disabilities act term," O'Connor said, "This act is one of those that did leave uncertainties in what it was Congress had in mind."[1]

In 2001 and 2002, the Supreme Court issued several milestone rulings involving persons with disabilities. These headline-making rulings will have a tremendous impact on how future policy is made in America. The cases are important because they illustrate the fact that disability activism alone cannot guarantee the rights of persons with disabilities, as well as the fact that old attitudes remain pervasive in society. The cases also are reflective of a Supreme Court that has continued to narrow the scope and coverage of the ADA.

Patricia Garrett began working as a nurse at the University of Alabama at Birmingham in 1977. She was a state employee who earned a master's degree as she worked her way up through the employment hierarchy. In June 1992 she was promoted to director of obstetric/gynecology neonatal services. Two years later, during a routine checkup, Garrett was diagnosed with breast cancer; she subsequently underwent surgery to remove her lymph nodes and later underwent extensive radiation and chemotherapy treatment. In March 1995 she was told that a subordinate would be taking over her position as director and that she would be transferred to a satellite location.

On her doctor's advice, Garrett took a four-month-long leave of absence under the 1993 Family and Medical Leave Act (FMLA), returning to work in July 1995. Initially, university officials agreed that she would continue in her previous position, but then they changed their minds, demoting her to a lower-paying position as a nurse manager. In response, she filed suit under the FMLA, Section 504 of the 1973 Rehabilitation Act, and the Americans with Disabilities Act of 1990. She alleged that she had been threatened repeatedly by the university with a transfer to a less-demanding job because of her treatment, that her supervisor had made negative comments about her illness, and that she was told that she would be permanently replaced unless she took sick leave. Garrett sought damages and equitable relief for discrimination, stating that her rights as an employee had been violated when she was demoted after taking sick leave. She also claimed that under the FMLA, she was required to be reinstated to an equivalent position, which the university refused to do.

To some observers, this episode might make an interesting case study in human resource management or employment law. The plaintiff has a compelling story, the university has power over its employees, and the state has the final decision-making capacity to determine how to handle the discrimination complaint. What makes Patricia Garrett's situation especially compelling, however, is that by filing suit she initiated a series of actions and decisions that may well determine the future of disability policy in the United States. It also serves as a test of the balancing of power between the federal government and the states.

The case was first heard in federal district court in 1998, where it was consolidated with another case, *Ash v. Alabama Department of Youth Services.*[2] The *Ash* case involved only the two disability statutes; it involved alleged discrimination against Milton Ash, who worked as a security officer in the Alabama Department of Youth Services. When Ash started work, he informed his supervisors that he had chronic asthma and that his doctor recommended that he avoid carbon monoxide and cigarette smoke. He asked that his duties be modified to minimize his exposure to these substances. He was later diagnosed with sleep apnea and requested, pursuant to his doctor's recommendation, that he be reassigned to daytime shifts to accommodate his condition. Ash's suit was based on the fact that the facility where he worked did not honor a no-smoking policy and failed to service its vehicles to keep toxic emissions from aggravating his condition. After he filed the suit, he then noticed that his performance evaluations were worse than those he had received on previous occasions.

The federal judge dismissed both suits (which had been filed separately) on summary judgment, on the grounds that the Eleventh Amendment to the Constitution grants sovereign immunity to states. The doctrine of sovereign immunity states that an individual cannot bring a suit against a government without its approval. The judge disposed of both cases, noting that neither party could file suit for money damages under the ADA.[3]

Both cases were then appealed to the Eleventh Circuit Court of Appeals.[4] In this venue, the U.S. Department of Justice intervened on the plaintiffs' behalf to defend the constitutionality of Congress's removal of Eleventh Amendment immunity, which had the effect of reversing the lower court's decision. The issue of whether a state is immune from suits by state employees asserting rights under federal law (such as the FMLA, the ADA, and the Rehabilitation Act) was being heard in several other circuit courts throughout the country at about the same time. A majority of the forty-three related Circuit Court decisions had found the ADA to be constitutional.

In the Eleventh Circuit, Chief Judge Roney, writing for the majority in a 2–1 decision, held that the state of Alabama was immune from suit under the provisions of the FMLA (which was at issue for Ms. Garrett), upholding what was generally called Eleventh Amendment immunity. In the case of legislation prohibiting discrimination against persons with disabilities, however, the court ruled that the U.S. Congress did have authority to pass laws that give citizens a right of action in federal court even when the state refuses to recognize that right. The opinion notes that in the ADA and the Rehabilitation Act, as well as in previous U.S. Supreme Court decisions, Congress explicitly found that persons with disabilities have suffered discrimination. This finding, the opinion notes, brings both statutes within the scope of appropriate legislation under the Equal Protection Clause as defined by the Supreme Court.

The state of Alabama chose to appeal, and the U.S. Supreme Court granted *certiorari* in the case on April 17, 2000. *Certiorari* was granted to resolve the split among the courts of appeal on the question of whether an individual may sue a state for monetary damages in federal court under the ADA.

The Supreme Court's decision to hear the *Garrett* case caused a firestorm of controversy among disability rights advocates, who for nearly ten years (since the signing of the ADA) had assumed that the question of whether disabled persons had been discriminated against was a given. To most of these advocates, the statute had made moot any remaining issues related to accessibility, equality, and opportunity, just as other civil rights statutes had done.

Seven states (Arkansas, Hawaii, Idaho, Nebraska, Nevada, Ohio, and Tennessee) supported Alabama's claim. Fourteen other states, in an *amicus* brief filed by the attorney general of Minnesota on behalf of his state, argued that the ADA's express abrogation of the states' Eleventh Amendment immunity was a proper exercise of congressional power to enforce the Equal Protection Clause.[5]

The lawyers representing Garrett and Ash contended that the ADA was a constitutionally appropriate measure to remedy past discrimination against persons with disabilities. The House and Senate committee hearings held prior to enactment of the statute found a lengthy history of discrimination in every state. For Congress, which held thirteen hearings specifically devoted to the constitutionality of the ADA, there was agreement that disabled persons experience "the most extreme isolation, unemployment, poverty, psychological abuse and physical deprivation experienced by any segment of our society."[6]

Subsequently, civil rights groups throughout the country began preparing *amici* briefs to be filed in support of Garrett and Ash; all told, more than a dozen briefs represented the diversity of the disability rights movement. One of the most comprehensive was a brief and compendium of state statutes, session laws, and constitutional provisions designed to show that Alabama (and other states) had a long history of discrimination against persons with disabilities even before the ADA was enacted. Much of the discrimination was employment related, although other documents confirmed discrimination in housing and zoning, forced sterilization, discrimination regarding the right to marry, and discrimination against parents with disabilities. Other evidence showed historical discrimination and interference with the rights of disabled persons to vote, to have equal access to the courts, and to travel, as well as discrimination against children with disabilities.[7]

In Alabama, for instance, the state code created a class of individuals defined as "mental inferiors or deficients, or feeble-minded."[8] Maryland decreed that any person "alleged to be a lunatic or insane" could be sent to a county or city almshouse.[9] Illinois law said that "no insane person or idiot shall be capable of contracting marriage."[10] Minnesota and Michigan agreed to authorize compulsory sterilization of mentally defective or insane institutional inmates,[11] and Mississippi made it unlawful to cohabit or attempt sexual intercourse with a feeble-minded female.[12] The compendium was created to underscore the federal government's argument that Congress had, indeed, considered past discrimination against persons with disabilities.

Another *amicus curiae* brief was filed by twenty organizations that included the American Civil Liberties Union, the Friends Committee on National Legislation, the National Urban League, and the NOW Legal Defense Fund. As with the federal government's argument, this brief noted that the central issue was whether the remedies afforded by the ADA are appropriate under the Fourteenth Amendment to remedy and deter unconstitutional state conduct. The brief argues, "The emphasis of the ADA is on eradicating prejudice and intentional discrimination, and protects only those with disabilities who in effect can demonstrate that they are similarly situated to others who seek or hold the job or service at issue. In fashioning a proportional response to the pervasive problem of disability discrimination, Congress recognized that the unique aspects of discrimination against individuals with disabilities require a different set of remedies provided in other civil rights statutes."[13]

A brief filed by the Southern Poverty Law Center represented twenty-seven disability, civil rights, family, and consumer organizations in Alabama, where the suit began. The "Alabama *Amici*" contended that the state's claim that it protects the rights of persons with disabilities was incorrect, documenting the state's "quaint habit of ignoring its responsibilities as a sovereign until faced with a federal court order."[14]

Even former president George Bush filed an *amicus* brief—an especially noteworthy action because he had supported the ADA and signed it into law in 1990. Although the brief focused more on Bush's accomplishments as president than legal argument, he did note that federal laws prior to the passage of the ADA "were like a patchwork quilt in need of repair. There were holes in the fabric, serious gaps in coverage that left persons with disabilities without adequate civil rights protections. To be effective in addressing the pervasive discrimination by public agencies, among others, the ADA needed to be cohesive, coordinated, and comprehensive."[15] Five current and two former members of Congress who were leaders in drafting the ADA filed briefs as well. Twelve constitutional law scholars with extensive experience in the study of the Fourteenth Amendment and the jurisdiction of the federal courts filed a brief urging the Supreme Court to defer to Congress' decision to remedy state violations of the constitutional rights of persons with disabilities.

On October 3, 2000, thousands of disability advocates from across the country came to Washington, D.C., in what was called "A March for Justice," on the grounds of the U.S. Capitol. Marca Bristo, chairperson of the National Council on Disability, said in a press briefing that day, "Why are we here? Why, before we realize the full promise of the law, are we debating its constitutionality? The lawyers here today can give you the legal answers to this question. People with disabilities, myself included, must give you the moral answer."[16] Although their presence was designed to draw support for the ADA and civil rights in general, it could not influence the nine justices of the Supreme Court, who heard oral arguments on October 11, 2000.[17]

Garrett and Ash were represented before the Court by Georgetown University law professor Michael Gottesman, along with U.S. Solicitor General Seth Waxman, representing the federal government. In their written brief, the focus was on Congress's power to enforce the Equal Protection Clause through legislation. In contrast to the circumstances of other civil rights statutes that the Supreme Court has found not applicable to state employers, prior to enactment of the ADA Congress received voluminous evidence of public-employer prejudice against people with disabilities. Gottesman and Waxman also argued that existing state laws were inadequate to address a pervasive pattern of employment discrimination. The U.S. Solicitor General's brief included the fact that although the ADA is designed to eradicate unconstitutional discrimination against individuals, it also preserves states' flexibility in the administration of their programs and services.

Alabama's case was argued by Jeffrey Sutton, who had been successful in a case the previous year that favored states' rights in the context of age discrimination. In that case, the Court ruled that Congress lacked the power to require states to pay damages for violations of the Age Discrimination in Employment Act.[18] Alabama argued that Congress did not act within its constitutional authority by subjecting the states to suits in federal court for money damages under the ADA.

The U.S. Supreme Court, in its 5–4 decision, ruled that employees of the state of Alabama may not recover money damages in employment discrimination suits against state governments under Title I of the ADA, under the provisions of the Eleventh Amendment.[19] In a footnote, the Court decided not to rule on the constitutionality of Title II, which has different remedial provisions from those in Title I. Chief Justice Rehnquist delivered the opinion of the Court, in which Justices O'Connor, Scalia,

Kennedy, and Thomas joined. Justice Kennedy filed a concurring opinion, in which Justice O'Connor joined. Justice Breyer filed a dissenting opinion, which was joined by Justices Stevens, Souter, and Ginsburg.

In the majority opinion, Rehnquist wrote that the Fourteenth Amendment to the Constitution does not require states to make special accommodations for disabled people, as long as their actions toward such individuals are rational.[20] The opinion states that the ADA's legislative record fails to show that Congress identified a history and pattern of irrational employment discrimination by the states against disabled people. The Court found only a half-dozen relevant incidents from the record that showed unconstitutional state action, noting that "these incidents taken together fall far short of even suggesting the pattern of unconstitutional discrimination." Instead, the Court noted that the statements included in the congressional hearings indicated that Congress targeted employment discrimination in the private sector.

The Court also determined that for the ADA to be held constitutional, there must be "congruence and proportionality between the injury to be prevented or remedied and the means adopted to that end."[21] Disposing of the argument that unconstitutional discrimination should extend not only to the states but also to local governments as state actors, the opinion used a footnote to acknowledge that by the time Congress enacted the ADA in 1990, every state had enacted a similar measure on its own. Several of the state laws, however, did not go as far as the ADA did in requiring accommodation—one of the major reasons disability advocates sought federal protection.

In their concurring opinion, Justices Kennedy and O'Connor acknowledged that prejudice against persons with disabilities does exist, stemming from indifference, insecurity, or malicious ill will. Kennedy writes, "I do not doubt that the Americans with Disabilities Act of 1990 will be a milestone on the path to a more decent, tolerant, progressive society." Yet he did not accept the argument that there had been a consistent violation of the equal protection standards of the Fourteenth Amendment, citing the lack of confirming judicial documentation.

Justice Breyer, in his dissenting opinion, disagreed with the majority
that there was no pattern of state discrimination. He stated that Congress
has compiled a vast legislative record documenting massive, society-wide
discrimination against persons with disabilities. "Congress reasonably
could have concluded that the remedy before us constitutes an 'appropriate' way to enforce this equal protection requirement. And that is all the
Constitution requires." Breyer created his own appendix of materials documenting 1,786 examples of state discrimination against disabled persons
and noted his belief that the ADA applies to local governments as well.
In effect, he accused the majority of ignoring the examples of discrimination by state governments found in the legislative record, rather than the
half-dozen on which the Court's opinion was based. Breyer cited as examples a case in which a zoo turned away children with Down Syndrome
because the zookeeper feared they would upset the chimpanzees and
another in which a state refused to hire a blind employee as director of an
agency for blind people even though he was the most qualified applicant.

In defending the reasonable accommodation requirement of the ADA,
the dissent asks rhetorically, "And what is wrong with a remedy that, in
response to unreasonable employer behavior, requires an employer to make
accommodations that are reasonable?" Breyer argues that whereas in the
past the Court deferred to Congress, in this case the Court abandoned that
principle; he wrote angrily, "The Court sounds the word of promise to the
ear but breaks it to the hope. . . . I doubt that today's decision serves any
constitutionally based federalism interest."

The decision would have made front-page headlines across the country
had it not been overshadowed by several other prominent stories that week
about Hillary Clinton's brother, the sinking of a Japanese fishing boat by
a U.S. submarine, and allegations regarding a U.S. intelligence officer pur-
ported to be spying for the Russians. Few media outlets paid more than
cursory attention to the ruling, which will be dissected in detail over the
next few years by legal and constitutional scholars.[22] One of the few daily
publications to comment on the case, the *Washington Post,* in an editorial
three days after the ruling was issued, perceived the case in terms of states'

rights rather than civil rights. "For in order to protect the states against disability discrimination suits, the court had to shackle further the federal power to ensure equal protection under the law."[23] An opinion piece by E. J. Dionne, Jr., characterized the case as part of the "rise of a new conservative judicial activism."[24] In the *New York Times*, the Court was said to have "carved out a new area of immunity for the states from the reach of federal civil rights law." The report was one of the few that recognized what the decision might portend, for other types of cases under the ADA and for other civil rights laws.[25]

A review of presidential press releases, White House briefings, and national media also revealed an interesting outcome: Neither President George W. Bush nor his father issued any comments on the *Garrett* decision in the two weeks following the ruling. The former president, who considered the ADA one of the most important legislative accomplishments of his administration, and his son, the current president—who campaigned on a pledge of "tearing down these barriers"—had nothing to say. Editorial pages were devoid of letters to the editor about the case, and it was mentioned only briefly on nightly newscasts.

For disability rights advocates and civil rights organizations across the country, however, the decision brought about stunned disbelief, especially over the Supreme Court's comments regarding a historic lack of evidence of discrimination against persons with disabilities. The National Council on Disability announced that it was "deeply troubled by the U.S. Supreme Court's rejection of substantial and powerful evidence of discriminatory treatment by state government that was carefully compiled and documented by the disability community and Congress." According to chairperson Marca Bristo, "We are deeply concerned that this ruling could be the slippery slope leading the 54 million Americans with disabilities back behind the closed doors that ADA promised to open. . . . The Supreme Court has put another obstacle in the path of people with disabilities."[26] Similarly, Jim Dixon of the National Organization on Disability stated, "This ruling is a blatant attack on the civil rights of persons with disabilities and may represent only the beginning of the erosion of the civil rights of all Americans."[27] In commenting on what it called a "disappointing decision," the American Civil Liberties Union, which also had filed an *amicus* brief, said the majority's conclusion that Congress overstepped its constitutional authority is both "inexplicable and wrong."[28]

Concerns were raised by the American Association of People with Disabilities; its president, Andrew Imparato, referred to the Court's "callous indifference to the impressive evidence of discrimination. . . . The U.S. Supreme Court is systematically turning the clock back on civil rights. The disability community is outraged that our highest court has chosen to weaken a law that is our ticket to full citizenship," he concluded.[29] Curtis Decker, executive director of the National Association of Protection and Advocacy Systems, noted, "The Supreme Court had before it myriad examples of discrimination. The question is, 'When is enough enough?'"[30]

Many organizations called on President George W. Bush to take action. The Arc of the United States, which represents persons with mental retardation and developmental disabilities, asked the president to continue to pursue disability employment cases and implored Congress to explore new legislation to restore the protections lost by the ruling. The language from the Arc was more optimistic, however, than that of other advocacy organizations; the group's president noted, "It is important for the public to understand that the ADA is not dead."[31] Disability rights attorney Harriet Johnson echoed those sentiments. "State employees facing disability discrimination in employment will be limited to state law and state court if they seek monetary damages. However, the decision very clearly leaves intact many key ADA principles."[32]

So where does American disability policy go from here? Just three weeks before the Supreme Court ruling in *Garrett*, President George W. Bush announced his New Freedom initiative—a measure that had been part of candidate Bush's campaign platform in 2000. The policy statement, which was then sent to Congress for action, acknowledged widespread discrimination against persons with disabilities. The president pledged to increase access to assistive and universally designed technology, to expand education opportunities for Americans with disabilities, to integrate them into the workforce, and to promote full access to community life. The initiative included specific requests for funding—including $1 billion to expand access to new technologies and $20 million to expand telecommuting—as well as implementation of existing statutes, such as the Ticket to Work and Work Incentives Improvement Act of 1999 and the Individuals with Disabilities Education Act. He also signed an executive order to create a National Commission on Mental Health Services to make recommendations for improving the nation's mental health service delivery system.[33]

A month earlier, the National Council on Disability, which makes recommendations on disability policy to the president, provided Bush with a series of transition recommendations for the new decade. The recommendations included a ten-point strategy that was based on a series of meetings in May 2000 to map out the elements of a ten-year program for more effective civil rights enforcement.[34]

Just five days after its ruling in *Garrett*, the Supreme Court decided that it would not get involved in the issue of whether disabled persons should be forced to pay some of the cost of their own accommodations. The Court declined to hear three cases from the circuit courts of appeals involving states that had levied fees for disabled parking placards.[35] The primary issue was the federal government's ban on any state surcharges to disabled people for providing special services. Almost lost in the shuffle, however, was a larger constitutional and ideological question, similar to that found in *Garrett*: whether Congress has authority to force states to take action (or not take action) under the ADA. Federal appeals courts have reached different conclusions about this issue, which is why the cases found their way to the U.S. Supreme Court.[36]

The Supreme Court also declined to hear a case that could have had an impact as significant as that in *Garrett*. In *United States v. Snyder*[37] a convicted burglar brought suit because he alleged Illinois prison officials did not make adequate accommodation for his partial blindness. John Walker's case arose under Title II of the ADA, which requires public entities to make their programs, services, and activities accessible to persons with disabilities. Walker argued that the state violated the statute by not responding to his request for books on tape, a very brightly lighted cell, and transfer to a less restrictive prison. The federal court agreed in part with the plaintiff's discrimination claim, but in 2000 the Seventh U.S. Circuit Court of Appeals dismissed the case on the grounds of state sovereignty under the Eleventh Amendment—the same argument used in *Garrett*. The appeals court held that Congress lacked authority to subject states to damage claims in federal court, despite the U.S. Justice Department's defense of the constitutionality of the ADA's application to the states. The Supreme Court agreed with Illinois prison officials' plea that it not step into the dispute.[37]

Although many Americans were oblivious to the *Garrett* case, few could ignore the headlines when the Supreme Court announced its decision in *PGA Tour, Inc. v. Martin* on May 29, 2001. Unlike the somewhat complex Title II issues raised in *Garrett,* the *Martin* case was fodder for media commentators as well as a situation with which many Americans could identify and about which they could form an opinion. Casey Martin's notoriety stemmed from a variety of factors. He had been a teammate of champion golfer Tiger Woods when the two attended Stanford University, and he had progressed to make the 1994 national collegiate championship team. He was supported in his public relations battle by Senators Bob Dole (R-KS) and Thomas Harkin (D-IA), who stood on the steps of the Capitol in Washington, D.C., with him, stating that rules and traditions must be changed. Although Martin also was supported by several disability rights groups, he faced the opposition of the U.S. Golf Association, the Ladies Professional Golf Association, and the men's professional tennis organization.

Martin sued the Professional Golf Association (PGA) under the ADA in November 1997. Martin was born with Klippel-Trenaunay-Weber Syndrome—an extremely rare, degenerative circulatory disorder that causes severe leg pain and makes walking for an extended period of time extremely difficult. He attempted to join the PGA and Nike tours by attending qualifying school, where golfers are permitted to use a cart in the first two of the school's three stages. Martin then asked to use a golf cart

for the third phase, and the PGA refused his request. He sued, alleging that
the nonprofit group failed to make its tournaments accessible to persons
with disabilities under Title III; he was successful in his arguments before
a district court.[38] He used a golf cart to qualify for the 1998 Nike Tour,
while the PGA appealed the decision to the Ninth Circuit Court of
Appeals.

Ruling a second time in favor of Martin in March 2000, the Circuit
Court noted that the PGA is not a private club and therefore is not exempt
from the provisions in the ADA, and golf courses are public accommodations covered by the statute. In addition, the court noted that allowing
Martin to use a golf cart is a reasonable accommodation that does not fundamentally alter the nature of the qualifying school, nor does it provide
him with an advantage over his competition.[39] Ironically, the day after the
Ninth Circuit's ruling was issued, the Seventh Circuit came to the opposite conclusion in the case of another disabled golfer, Fred Olinger.[40]

In July 2000 the PGA appealed to the U.S. Supreme Court, arguing
that Title III was not applicable and that, in fact, Martin was an "enter-
tainer" who could only file job-related claims of discrimination. The peti-
tioners also noted that by allowing Martin to use a cart, the PGA would
be waiving the "outcome affecting" requirement that all tournament participants walk the golf course.

In its 7–2 ruling affirming the Ninth Circuit's decision, the Supreme
Court highlighted Martin's athletic prowess, calling him a "talented golfer"
who still walked about 25 percent of the course over a five-hour period.
Justice Stevens, writing for the majority, also criticized the PGA for failing
to consider Martin's "personal circumstances" in deciding whether to
accommodate his disability—an interpretation that requires modification
on a case-by-case basis. That fact, the opinion notes, is consistent with congressional intent to "give individualized attention to the handful of requests
that it [the PGA] might receive from talented or disabled athletes."[41]
Ironically, Justice Stevens's majority opinion refers to Congress's intent "to
remedy widespread discrimination against disabled individuals." Yet in
Garrett, the majority decided that discrimination does not actually exist

and that the historical record and compelling need referred to by Stevens do not demonstrate a pattern of discrimination.

Commentary on the *Martin* decision was predictable. Disability organizations praised the Court for its decision but were angry with coverage of the case and the way it was portrayed by many sports columnists. *Ragged Edge* magazine criticized several publications for emphasizing the fact that Martin's situation was an isolated one and that this case focused on an individual's medical problems rather than civil rights and discrimination.[42] Trying to put a different spin on the outcome, the National Organization on Disability said that the case "has enhanced the nation's awareness and understanding of the ADA. This legislation is the core of civil rights for people with disabilities."[43] Cable News Network's Charles Bierbauer emphasized the need to make individualized judgments about what kind of accommodation is needed, adding that it did not mean everyone would be allowed to play on the PGA Tour.[44] *The Sporting News*, in an earlier column, noted that golfer Jack Nicklaus said that riding a cart creates "an uneven playing field for Martin." In response, the magazine's Dave Kindred commented, "To hear these elitist whiners, you'd think Martin has asked to hit from women's tees or to count only every third stroke. A dying leg has already made the playing field uneven for Casey Martin."[45] The case generated humorous speculation about accommodations for blind bowlers and football place kickers or how golfers with bad backs also might seek to be declared disabled. Several commentators used the analogy of Justice Scalia, who compared Martin's situation to giving a Little League baseball player with attention deficit disorder four strikes instead of three because it was 25 percent more difficult for that player to hit a pitched ball.

For many observers, however, Casey Martin was more symbolic of the legal system gone haywire than a blow for civil rights. The justices seemed clear that they were making an exception in Martin's case, that they expected only a handful of requests for modifications, and that the golfer's talent somehow made up for the fact that he was disabled. Justice Scalia's dissent (which Justice Thomas joined) speaks of "benevolent compassion" for Martin and terms "silly" the entire question of whether walking is a fundamental aspect of golf. He goes further to allege that the ruling will produce numerous cases in which an individual requests special treatment—"a rich source of lucrative litigation." Scalia refers to the ruling as "this Court's Kafkaesque determination," "its Alice in Wonderland determination," and its "Animal Farm determination"—as if there were no legal grounds for the decision at all.[46]

President George W. Bush's silence on the *Garrett* and *Martin* cases is telling. It indicates a chief executive who recognizes the political wisdom of not commenting on a statute his father signed into law that was found unconstitutional, as well as a president who is cognizant of the forces of public opinion and media coverage. The president is not likely to take up the mantle of leadership for the civil rights of disabled persons as his father did. As governor of Texas, he was not a strong supporter of disability issues, according to advocates in that state who repeatedly tried to meet with him. Texas members of ADAPT had protested at the Governor's mansion for days when Bush signed on to the states' rights brief in the *Olmstead* case when it was before the U.S. Supreme Court.[47]

Bush marked the eleventh anniversary of the signing of the ADA with a radio address to the nation on July 28, 2001. He noted that he was proud that his father had signed the bill and said that citizens with disabilities had gained greater access to public places, homes, transportation, employment, and travel. He also noted that some barriers remain and referred to the New Freedom Initiative he had proposed a few months earlier. He called on Congress "to provide the resources we need to fully fund the New Freedom Initiative and fulfill the promise of the ADA."[48]

The Supreme Court returned to its pattern of narrowing the definition of disability in its January 8, 2002, ruling against Ella Williams, an automobile assembly-line employee with carpal tunnel syndrome. Her job required her to use pneumatic tools, and the repetitive motion led to the painful muscle injuries. Williams was reassigned to another position as a vehicle paint inspector—a job that no longer exacerbated her condition. Later, however, she was assigned to do other manual tasks, and the pain returned. She asked to go back to her job as a paint inspector as an accommodation under the ADA. She stopped going to work and was fired. In *Toyota Motor Mfg. v. Williams,* 122 S.Ct. 681, a unanimous Supreme Court agreed that because Williams was still able to perform a major life activity (tasks such as brushing her teeth and bathing) when she requested the accommodation, she was not protected by the ADA as a disabled person.[49]

"If Congress intended everyone with a physical impairment that precluded the performance of some isolated, unimportant or particularly difficult manual task to qualify as disabled, the number of disabled Americans would surely have been much higher," Justice Sandra Day O'Connor wrote. "The manual tasks unique to any particular job are not necessarily important parts of most people's lives." She asserted that the impairment must be permanent or long term. "It is insufficient for individuals attempting to prove disability status under this test to merely submit evidence of a medical diagnosis of an impairment."[50]

Legal scholars are just beginning to analyze rulings such as that in *Williams,* with one review noting that there is uncertainty about the impact of the decision. "While some employers and defense attorneys applaud the ruling, predicting that it will limit employee demands and litigation, others expressed concern that the individualized assessment standard will result in many cases continuing to jury trials rather than being resolved by way of summary judgment. Some opponents of the ADA-narrowing result in this case fault Congress rather than the Supreme Court and characterize the decision as a fair interpretation of an 'imprecise law.'"[51]

Professor Ruth O'Brien, commenting on the *Williams* ruling, said, "She's trapped in another variation on the 'Catch 22' in the Supreme Court's interpretation of the Americans with Disabilities Act. . . . Although Williams is so disabled that she cannot work without accommodations, she is not disabled enough to receive protection under the ADA. The Supreme Court is presenting Williams and the 600,000 workers who lose work time every year because of similar injuries with a dilemma that is perverse and precarious."[52]

On April 29, 2002, the Supreme Court narrowed even further the boundaries of the ADA in one of its rare rulings on what constitutes undue hardship under the law. Robert Barnett, a former U.S. Airways customer service agent with back problems, asked to be transferred to a job in the company's mailroom. A year later, Barnett was replaced by a worker with more seniority, and he filed suit, arguing that the airline should carve out a disability exception to seniority to accommodate him. In questioning the lawyers in the case, the justices seemed to hint that they were unpersuaded by Barnett's request for an exception.[53]

The divided opinion in *U.S. Airways v. Barnett* (No. 00-1250) shows that the justices had mixed feelings about their reasons for ruling against Barnett; they remanded the decision back to the lower court to allow him to pursue his case. Justice Breyer, who delivered the opinion of the Court, noted that traditionally the issues of reasonable accommodation and undue hardship provisions were decided on their face. This requires the employer to show special circumstances that demonstrate undue hardship in a particular case. The Court agreed that Barnett could still attempt to demonstrate the special circumstances of his case, with the justices even making suggestions on how that might be accomplished. The opinion adds that the plaintiff has the burden of showing special circumstances and must explain why, in the particular case, an exception to the seniority system can constitute a reasonable accommodation even though in the ordinary case it cannot.[54]

The justices narrowed the applicability of the ADA one more time in the 2001–2002 term in its June 10, 2002, ruling in *Chevron U.S.A. Inc. v. Echazabal* (No. 00-1406). Mario Echazabal, who worked at a Chevron oil refinery for several years under contract, applied directly to Chevron for a job. He was hired, contingent on passing a physical examination. He was diagnosed with hepatitis C, and Chevron not only withdrew its job offer but told contractors they could no longer employ him at the facility. Echazabal sued the company for discrimination under the ADA, claiming that an employer cannot refuse to hire an individual because of concerns that a disability will pose a direct threat to his own health or safety.

Echazabal's attorney, Larry Minsky, told a reporter that "an employer must allow an employee, or applicant in this case, to perform a job if the employee is fully informed, accepts the risk of a job, and says, 'I can do it.'"[55] Chevron argued that under an EEOC regulation, an employer could bar an employee with a disability from the workplace by showing that the job would pose a direct threat to his health. In its unanimous decision, the Supreme Court ruled against Echazabal, allowing the EEOC regulation to stand in the face of the ADA. The justices declined to hear a similar case in May 2002 involving the appeal of a dental hygienist who was removed from his job when his employer learned that he had HIV. A district court had ruled against the employee because there was a "sound, theoretical" possibility of transmission that posed a direct threat.

The U.S. Chamber of Commerce, whose legal arm had filed an *amicus* brief in the *Echazabal* case, called the decision "a major victory for the business community." The brief had argued that an employer might also be potentially liable under the Occupational Safety and Health Act of 1970 if an employer hired an employee knowing that the job posed a direct threat to the individual's own health and safety.[56] The National Council on Disability called the ruling "paternalistic. . . . We are so appalled by the decision, it is as if the Supreme Court justices read a different law than we did. We wouldn't think of doing this to any other group of people."[57]

The 2001–2002 term ended with a bittersweet victory for disabled rights activists. In one of its final decisions for the session, the justices ruled in *Atkins v. Virginia* (No. 00-8452) that executions of mentally retarded criminals are cruel and unusual punishments prohibited by the Eighth Amendment. The case involved a Virginia inmate, Daryl Renard Atkins, who had been convicted of shooting a man in 1996. Atkins' attorneys argued that he has an IQ of 59 and that he had never been able to live on his own or hold a job. In a 6–3 decision, the Court found that although mentally retarded persons frequently know the difference between right and wrong and are competent to stand trial, by definition they have diminished capacities that reduce their personal culpability. The majority opinion by Justice Stevens noted that mentally retarded defendants face a special risk of wrongful execution because they may unwittingly confess to crimes they did not commit, they may be unable to provide their attorneys with meaningful assistance, they tend to be poor witnesses, and their demeanor "may create an unwarranted impression of lack of remorse for their crimes."[58]

The Court was not willing to forego punishment altogether, nor did it address the issue of the constitutionality of the death penalty. The Court did defer to legislative consensus that the death penalty was inappropriate for mentally retarded offenders, citing shifts in public attitudes since the Court ruled in 1989 that the practice was constitutional. By 2002, the number of states that had outlawed the death penalty for mentally retarded offenders had risen from only two to eighteen. Justice Stevens wrote, "It is not so much the number of these states that is significant, but the consistency of the direction of the change. . . . The practice . . . has become unusual, and it is fair to say that a national consensus has developed against it."[59]

The ruling was heralded by advocates for persons who are mentally retarded. James Ellis, Atkins' attorney and past president of the American Association on Mental Retardation (AAMR), argued that public opinion on executing mentally retarded defendants had changed, even among those who support the death penalty: "They are deeply disturbed by the prospect that people with mental retardation could face execution." The executive director of AAMR said, "I am deeply grateful that the Supreme Court justices have put an end to this barbaric practice of killing persons who do not have the full intellectual capacity to understand the crime they committed. This is an important day for disability advocates and for our country."[60]

CONCLUSION

Despite the victory in *Atkins*, some observers question whether disability rights groups will be able once again to muster the political clout that brought about the signing of the ADA in 1990. Many of the statute's original advocates have died or are growing old or tired from decades of legislative and judicial warfare, and there are fewer new recruits to take their places. Some activists are starting to regroup at the state level—similar to tactics used by women's groups after they failed to win passage of the Equal Rights Amendment. In 2001, for example, California's Prudence K. Popick Act established protections that are intentionally stronger than those of the ADA. The law includes in its definition of a disability conditions not specifically covered in the federal statute—such as clinical depression, heart disease, and epilepsy—and does not require that a person's major life activities be substantially limited by excluding the word "substantially." Rhode Island, responding to the *Sutton* ruling in June 1999, amended its constitution to protect persons with disabilities whose conditions were mitigated by medication or assistive technology. Advocates will end up, however, with a situation similar to what they faced in the pre-ADA years: a patchwork of different definitions and regulations rather than a national antidiscrimination law.

The ADA is not dead, but it has been wounded by the courts and almost ignored by a Congress and president that have moved on to other causes, other issues. More important, it is clear that the courts' attack on the ADA is not yet over, and disability rights advocates fear that the conservative Supreme Court will continue to rule against employees as it did in the *Garrett* case. O'Brien's analysis of the role of the courts in workplace lawsuits sums up the issue: "Acting as state experts, the federal court judges control what each individual should receive, be it a reasonable accommodation or termination as a result of exposing a limiting, but not substantially limiting, impairment to his or her employer."[61]

O'Brien goes on to examine the courts' role as a gatekeeper—an activity usually performed by administrative agencies or an executive department that has been given the authority to implement a public policy or program. "The situation will not change if the courts continue protecting employers from the burden of even facing, let alone losing, suits from employees or prospective employees who request reasonable accommodations."[62]

There is little that disability rights activists can do, however, when these controversies reach the judicial arena. The building of coalitions, demonstrations, letter writing, and legislative maneuvering that marked the successful passage of the ADA in 1990 can be overruled in a single decision by justices far removed from the rest of the political system. In such a partisan political environment, traditional tactics are of limited value at best.

Meanwhile, the symbolic struggle continues. On January 10, 2001, President Bill Clinton unveiled a life-size statue of President Franklin Delano Roosevelt in Washington, D.C.'s West Potomac Park. Such events are not especially newsworthy, but this was no ordinary bronze monument. When Roosevelt had been a young man, he contracted polio, and for the rest of his life (and with the assistance of the media and fellow politicians) he hid his disability from the public. There are only four photographs of FDR in his wheelchair. He worried that world leaders and the American people would perceive him as being weak. The new statue at the FDR National Memorial, however, portrays Roosevelt in a wheelchair he designed for himself. The statue was built not with public funds but with donations from the public and the National Organization on Disability, which gathered support for a "real" portrayal of the president. One of Roosevelt's quotations on the passageway to room three of the memorial exemplifies what still needs to be done to ensure equality for persons with disabilities: "We must scrupulously guard the civil rights and civil liberties of all citizens, whatever their background. We must remember that any oppression, any injustice, any hatred is a wedge designed to attack our civilization."[63]

APPENDIX A

Suggestions for Further Research

ACCESSIBILITY AND ARCHITECTURAL BARRIERS

Evan Terry Associates. 1993. *Americans with Disabilities Act Facilities Compliance: A Practical Guide.* New York: John Wiley.

Hablutzel, Nancy, and Brian McMahon, eds. 1992. *Americans with Disabilities Act: Access and Accommodations.* Orlando, Fla.: Paul M. Deutsch Press.

Johnson, Mary, and others, eds. 1992. *People with Disabilities Explain It All for You: Your Guide to the Public Accommodations Requirements of the Americans with Disabilities Act.* Louisville, Ky.: Advocado Press.

Lebovich, William L. 1993. *Design for Dignity: Accessible Environments for People with Disabilities.* New York: John Wiley.

Null, Roberta, with Kenneth F. Cherry. 1998. *Universal Design: Creative Solutions for ADA Compliance.* Belmont, Calif.: Professional Publications.

Rehabilitation Engineering Center. 1990. *Architectural Accessibility Resources.* Washington, D.C.: National Rehabilitation Hospital.

Stanfield, Edward, and G. Scott Danforth. 1999. *Enabling Environments: Measuring the Impact of Environment on Disability and Rehabilitation.* New York: Plenum.

U.S. Department of Health and Human Services. 1996. *Opening Our Doors and Removing the Barriers.* Washington, D.C.: U.S. Department of Health and Human Services.

Welch, Polly, ed. 1995. *Strategies for Teaching Universal Design.* Boston: Adaptive Environments Center.

AMERICANS WITH DISABILITIES ACT OF 1990: GENERAL

Anderson, Robert Carl, ed. 1996. *A Look Back: The Birth of the Americans with Disabilities Act.* New York: Haworth.

Bishop, Peter C., and Augustus J. Jones, Jr. 1993. "Implementing the Americans with Disabilities Act of 1990: Assessing the Variables of Success." *Public Administration Review* 53 (March/April): 121–28.

Burgdorf, Robert L., Jr. 1991. "The Americans with Disabilities Act: Analysis and Implications of a Second Generation Civil Rights Statute." *Harvard Civil Rights-Civil Liberties Law Review* 26 (summer): 413–522.

Burkhauser, Richard V. 1990. "Morality on the Cheap: The Americans with Disabilities Act." *Cato Review of Business and Government* 13, no. 2: 47–56.

Cook, Timothy M. 1991. "The Americans with Disabilities Act: The Move to Integration." *Temple Law Review* 64: 393–469.

D'Agostino, Thomas. 1997. *Defining "Disability" Under the ADA: 1997 Update.* Horsham, Pa.: LRP Publications.

Dar, Tatiana. 1997. "Blueprint for Segregation." *Mainstream* (June/July), 31–33.

Gostin, Lawrence O., and Henry A. Beyer, eds. 1993. *Implementing the Americans with Disabilities Act: Rights and Responsibilities for All Americans.* Baltimore: Paul H. Brookes.

Harkin, Tom. 1990. "Our Newest Civil Rights Law: The Americans with Disabilities Act." *Trial* 56 (December): 56–61.

Johnson, William G. 1997. *The Americans with Disabilities Act: Social Contract or Special Privilege?* Thousand Oaks, Calif.: Sage.

Johnson, William G., and Marjorie Baldwin. 1993. "The Americans with Disabilities Act: Will It Make a Difference?" *Policy Studies Journal* 21, no. 4: 775–88.

Jones, N. L. 1991. "Overview and Essential Requirements of the Americans with Disabilities Act." *Temple Law Review* 64, no. 2: 471–98.

Jones, Timothy L. 1993. *The Americans with Disabilities Act: A Review of Best Practices.* New York: American Management Association.

Kopelman, Loretta M. 1996. "Ethical Assumptions and Ambiguities in the Americans with Disabilities Act." *Journal of Medicine and Philosophy* 21: 187–208.

Montanaro, Lisa A. 1995. "The Americans with Disabilities Act: Will the Court Get the Hint?" *Pace Law Review* 15: 621–83.

National Council on Disability. 1993. *ADA Watch: Year One*. Washington, D.C.: National Council on Disability.

———. 1995. *The Americans with Disabilities Act: Ensuring Equal Access to the American Dream*. Washington, D.C.: National Council on Disability.

———. 1997. *Equality of Opportunity: The Making of the Americans with Disabilities Act*. Washington, D.C.: National Council on Disability.

Parmet, Wendy E. 1990. "Discrimination and Disability: The Challenges of the ADA." *Law, Medicine and Health Care* 18: 331–44.

Percy, Stephen L. 1993. "The ADA: Expanding Mandates for Disability Rights." *Intergovernmental Perspective* 19 (winter): 11–14.

———. 1993. "ADA, Disability Rights, and Evolving Regulatory Federalism." *Publius* 23 (fall): 87–105.

———. 2001. "Challenges and Dilemmas in Implementing the Americans with Disabilities Act: Lessons from the First Decade." *Policy Studies Journal* 29, no. 4: 633–40.

Pfeiffer, David. 1994. "The Americans with Disabilities Act: Costly Mandates or Civil Rights." *Disability and Society* 9, no. 4: 533–42.

Rioux, Marcia H., Cameron Crawford, and Jane Anweiler. 2001. "Undue Hardship and Reasonable Accommodation: The View from the Court." *Policy Studies Journal* 29, no. 4: 641–48.

Spechler, Jay W. 1996. *Reasonable Accommodation: Profitable Compliance with the Americans with Disabilities Act*. Delray Beach, Fla.: St. Lucie Press.

U.S. Department of Justice. 2000. *Enforcing the ADA: Looking Back on a Decade of Progress*. Washington, D.C.: U.S. Department of Justice.

Watson, Sara. 1994. "Applying Theory to Practice: A Prospective and Prescriptive Analysis of the Implementation of the Americans with Disabilities Act." *Journal of Disability Policy Studies* 5, no. 1: 1–23.

West, Jane, ed. 1991. *The Americans with Disabilities Act: From Policy to Practice*. New York: Milbank Memorial Fund.

———. 1994. *Federal Implementation of the Americans with Disabilities Act, 1991–1994*. New York: Milbank Memorial Fund.

———. 1996. *Implementing the Americans with Disabilities Act*. Cambridge, Mass.: Blackwell.

Wilson, Edwina A. 1992–1993. "Practical Considerations for Compliance Under the Americans with Disabilities Act." *Gonzaga Law Review* 28, no. 2: 265–90.

AMERICANS WITH DISABILITIES ACT OF 1990: STATE AND LOCAL GOVERNMENTS

Byers, Keith A. 1997. "No One Is Above the Law When It Comes to the ADA and the Rehabilitation Act—Not Even Federal, State, or Local Law Enforcement Agencies." *Loyola Los Angeles Law Review* 977 (April): 30.

Coleman, John J., and Marcel L. DeBruge. 1993. "A Practitioner's Introduction to ADA Title II." *Alabama Law Review* 45 (fall): 55.

McCarty, Kathryn S. 1991. *Complying with the ADA of 1990: Local Officials Guide*. Washington, D.C.: National League of Cities.

Parry, J. "State and Local Government Services Under the ADA: Nondiscrimination on the Basis of Disability." *Mental and Physical Disability Law Reporter* 15: 615–21.

Slack, James D. 1996. "Workplace Preparedness and the Americans with Disabilities Act: Lessons from Municipal Governments' Management of HIV/AIDS." *Public Administration Review* 56, no. 2 (March–April): 159–67.

———. 1998. *HIV/AIDS and the Public Workplace*. Tuscaloosa: University of Alabama Press.

Switzer, Jacqueline Vaughn. 2001. "Local Government Implementation of the Americans with Disabilities Act." *Policy Studies Journal* 29, no. 4: 654–62.

Wolfe, Ann M. 1989. *Disabled Persons: State Laws Concerning Accessibility and Discrimination*. Washington, D.C.: Congressional Research Service.

CHILDREN

Ayrault, Evelyn West. 2001. *Beyond a Physical Disability: The Person Within*. New York: Continuum.

Batshaw, Mark L. ed. 1997. *Children with Disabilities*. Baltimore: Paul H. Brookes.

Committee on Children with Disabilities. 1996. "The Role of the Pediatrician in Implementing the Americans with Disabilities Act." *Pediatrics* 98, no. 1: 116–18.

Doggett, Libby, and Jill George. 1993. *All Kids Count*. Arlington, Tex.: The Arc.

Gleidman, John, and William Roth. 1980. *The Unexpected Minority:*

Handicapped Children in America. New York: Harcourt Brace Jovanovich.

Morgan, Sharon R. 1987. *Abuse and Neglect of Handicapped Children.* Boston: Little, Brown, and Co.

Powers, Michael D., ed. 2000. *Children with Autism: A Parents' Guide.* Bethesda, Md.: Woodbine House.

Thompson, Charlotte. 2000. *Raising a Handicapped Child.* New York: Oxford University Press.

Westcott, Helen L. 1996. *This Far and No Further: Toward Ending the Abuse of Disabled Children.* Birmingham, Ala.: Venture Press.

Deafness and Deaf Culture

Baker, Charlotte, and Carol Padden. 1978. *American Sign Language: A Look at Its History, Structure, and Community.* Silver Spring, Md.: T. J. Publishers.

Baldwin, Stephen C. 1993. *Pictures in the Air: The Story of the National Theatre of the Deaf.* Washington, D.C.: Gallaudet University Press.

Baynton, Douglas. 1996. *Forbidden Signs: American Culture and the Campaign against Sign Language.* Chicago: University of Chicago Press.

Bragg, Lois, ed. 2001. *Deaf World: A Historical Reader and Primary Sourcebook.* New York: New York University Press.

Cohen, Leah H. 1994. *Train Go Sorry: Inside a Deaf World.* Boston: Houghton Mifflin.

Groce, Nora E. 1985. *Everyone Here Spoke Sign Language.* Cambridge, Mass.: Harvard University Press.

Lane, Harlan. 1984. *When the Mind Hears: A History of the Deaf.* New York: Random House.

Tucker, Bonnie P. 1997. "The ADA and Deaf Culture: Contrasting Precepts, Conflicting Results." *Annals of the American Academy of Political and Social Science* 549 (January): 24–36.

Van Cleve, John V., and Barry A. Crouch. 1989. *A Place of Their Own: Creating the Deaf Community in America.* Washington, D.C.: Gallaudet University Press.

Wilcox, Sherman, ed. 1989. *American Deaf Culture.* Burstonsville, Md.: Linstok Press.

DEMOGRAPHICS

Gleason, John J. 1989. *Special Education in Context: An Ethnographic Study of Persons with Developmental Disabilities.* Cambridge: Cambridge University Press.

Hoffman, Susan T., and Inez Fitzgerald Storch, eds. 1991. *Disability in the United States: A Portrait from National Data.* New York: Springer Publishing Company.

International Center for the Disabled (ICD). 1986. *The ICD Survey of Disabled Americans: Bringing Disabled Americans into the Mainstream.* New York: International Center for the Disabled.

La Plante, Mitch. 1991. "The Demographics of Disability." *Milbank Quarterly* 69: 55–80.

———. 1991. "Disability in Basic Life Activities across the Life Span." *Disability Statistics Report* 1: 1–42.

Wolfe, Barbara, and Robert H. Haveman. 1990. "Trends in the Prevalence of Disability 1962–1984." *Milbank Quarterly* 68, no. 1: 53–80.

Zola, Irving K. 1993. "Disability Statistics: What We Count and What It Tells Us." *Journal of Disability Policy Studies* 4, no. 4: 9–39.

DISABILITY POLICY: GENERAL

Batavia, Andrew I. 1993. "Relating Disability Policy to Broader Public Policy: Understanding the Concept of 'Handicap.'" *Policy Studies Journal* 21, no. 4: 735–39.

Berkowitz, Edward D. 1987. *Disabled Policy: America's Programs for the Handicapped.* Cambridge: Cambridge University Press.

———. 1992. "Disabled Policy: A Personal Postscript." *Journal of Disability Policy Studies* 3, no. 1: 1–16.

Berkowitz, Monroe, William G. Johnson, and Edward H. Murphy. 1976. *Public Policy Toward Disability.* New York: Praeger.

Bickenbach, Jerome Edward. 1993. *Physical Disability and Social Policy.* Toronto: University of Toronto Press.

Bowe, Frank. 1978. *Handicapping America: Barriers to Disabled People.* Baltimore: Paul H. Brookes.

Bryan, Willie V. 1996. *In Search of Freedom: How Persons with Disabilities Have Been Disenfranchised from the Mainstream of American Society.* Springfield, Ill.: C. C. Thomas.

Burkhauser, Richard V., and others. 1993. "How People with Disabilities Fare When Public Policies Change." *Journal of Policy Analysis and Management* 12, no. 2: 251–69.

Campbell, Jane, and Mike Oliver. 1996. *Disability Politics: Understanding Our Past, Changing Our Future.* New York: Routledge.

DeJong, Gerben, and Andrew I. Batavia, 1990. "The Americans with Disabilities Act and the Current State of U.S. Disability Policy." *Journal of Disability Policy* 1, no. 3 (fall): 65–82.

———. 1991. "The Americans with Disabilities Act: Definitions of Disability." *Labor Lawyer* 7: 11–26.

Hahn, Harlan. 1985. "Disability Policy and the Problem of Discrimination." *American Behavioral Scientist* 28: 293–318.

———. 1985. "Toward a Politics of Disability: Definitions, Disciplines, and Policy." *Social Science Journal* 22 (October): 87–105.

———. 1993. "The Potential Impact of Disability Studies on Political Science (as Well as Vice Versa)." *Policy Studies Journal* 21, no. 4: 740–51.

Howards, Irving, Henry P. Brehm, and Saad Z. Nagi. 1980. *Disability: From Social Problem to Federal Program.* New York: Praeger.

Johnson, William G. 1997. "The Future of Disability Policy: Benefit Payments or Civil Rights?" *Annals of the American Academy of Political and Social Science* (January): 160–72.

Kaye, H. Stephen. 1998. *Is the Status of Persons with Disabilities Improving?* Washington, D.C.: U.S. Department of Education.

———. 2001. *Disability Watch,* vol. 2. Oakland, Calif.: Disability Rights Advocates.

National Council on Disability. 1996. *Achieving Independence: The Challenge for the 21st Century.* Washington, D.C.: National Council on Disability.

National Council on the Handicapped. 1986. *Toward Independence: An Assessment of Federal Laws and Programs Affecting Persons with Disabilities.* Washington, D.C.: National Council on the Handicapped.

Percy, Stephen L. 1989. *Disability, Civil Rights, and Public Policy: The Politics of Implementation.* Tuscaloosa: University of Alabama Press.

———. 1993. "Challenges and Dilemmas in Implementing Disability Rights Policies." *Journal of Disability Policy Studies* 4, no. 1 (summer): 41–63.

President's Committee on Employment of People with Disabilities. 1994. *Operation People First.* Washington, D.C.: President's Committee on Employment of People with Disabilities.

Scotch, Richard K. 1994. "Understanding Disability Policy: Varieties of Analysis." *Policy Studies Journal* 22, no. 1: 171–75.

———. 2001. *From Good Will to Civil Rights: Transforming Federal Disability Policy,* 2d ed. Philadelphia: Temple University Press.

Stone, Deborah. 1984. *The Disabled State.* Philadelphia: Temple University Press.

U.S. Advisory Commission on Intergovernmental Relations. 1989. *Disability Rights Mandates: Federal and State Compliance with Employment Protections and Architectural Barrier Removal.* Washington, D.C.: U.S. Government Printing Office.

U.S. Commission on Civil Rights. 1980. *Civil Rights Issues of Handicapped Americans: Public Policy Implications.* Washington, D.C.: U.S. Commission on Civil Rights.

DISABILITY RIGHTS MOVEMENT

Barnartt, Sharon, and John B. Christiansen. 1995. *Deaf President Now! The 1988 Revolution at Gallaudet University.* Washington, D.C.: Gallaudet University Press, 1995.

Charlton, James. 1998. *Nothing about Us without Us: Disability Oppression and Empowerment.* Berkeley: University of California Press.

Driedger, Diane. 1989. *The Last Civil Rights Movement.* New York: St. Martin's Press.

Fleischer, Doris James, and Frieda Zames. 2001. *The Disability Rights Movement: From Charity to Confrontation.* Philadelphia: Temple University Press.

Golden, Marilyn. 1996. "Damn Straight We're a Real Movement!" *Disability Rag and Resource* 17, no. 2 (March–April): 1, 4–5, 15.

Johnson, Mary, and Barrett Shaw, eds. 2001. *To Ride the Public's Buses: The Fight that Built a Movement.* Louisville, Ky.: Advocado Press.

Little, Jan. 1996. *If It Weren't for the Honor—I'd Rather Have Walked: Previously Untold Tales of the Journey to the ADA.* Cambridge, Mass.: Brookline Books.

Longmore, Paul. 2001. *The New Disability History: American Perspectives*. New York: New York University Press.

Matson, Floyd. 1990. *Walking Alone and Marching Together: A History of the Organized Blind Movement in the United States, 1940–1990*. Baltimore: National Federation of the Blind.

McGuire, Jean Flatley. 1994. "Organizing from Diversity in the Name of Community: Lessons from the Disability Civil Rights Movement." *Policy Studies Journal* 22: 119.

Pelka, Fred. 1997. *The ABC-CLIO Companion to the Disability Rights Movement*. Santa Barbara, Calif.: ABC-CLIO.

Pfeiffer, David. 1993. "Overview of the Disability Movement: History, Legislative Record, and Political Implications." *Policy Studies Journal* 21, no. 4: 724–34.

Scotch, Richard K. 1988. "Disability as a Basis of a Social Movement: Advocacy and the Politics of Definition." *Journal of Social Issues* 44, no. 1: 173–88.

———. 1989. "Politics and Policy in the History of the Disability Rights Movement." *Milbank Quarterly* 67: 380–400.

Shapiro, Joseph. 1993. *No Pity: The Story of the Disability Rights Movement and How It Is Changing America*. New York: Random House.

Shaw, Barrett. 1994. *Ragged Edge: The Disability Experience from the Pages of the First Fifteen Years of the Disability Rag*. Louisville, Ky.: Advocado Press.

Watson, Sara, and Bonnie O'Day. 1996. "Movement Leadership." *Disability Studies Quarterly* 16, no. 1 (winter): 26–30.

Employment and Rehabilitation

Albrecht, Gary. 1992. *The Disability Business: Rehabilitation in America*. New York: Russell Sage.

Baldwin, Marjorie L. 1997. "Can the ADA Achieve Its Employment Goals?" *Annals of the Academy of Political and Social Science* 549 (January): 37–52.

Berkowitz, Edward, and Monroe Berkowitz. 1990. "Labor Force Participation among Disabled Persons." *Research in Labor Economics* 11: 181–200.

Berkowitz, Monroe, and Ann Hill, eds. 1986. *Disability and the Labor Market: Economic Problems, Policies, and Programs*. Ithaca, N.Y.: ILR Press.

Blanck, Peter David, ed. 2001. *Employment, Disability, and the ADA*. Chicago: Northwestern University Press.

Bonnie, Richard J., and John Monahan, eds. 1997. *Mental Disorder, Work Disability, and the Law*. Chicago: University of Chicago Press.

Braddock, David. 1994. *The Glass Ceiling and Persons with Disabilities*. Chicago: Institute on Disability and Human Development.

Brandfield, Julie. 1990. "Undue Hardship: Title I of the Americans with Disabilities Act." *Fordham Law Review* 59, no. 1: 113–33.

Burgdorf, Robert L. Jr. 1995. *Disability Discrimination in Employment Law*. Washington, D.C.: Bureau of National Affairs.

Burkhauser, Richard V. 1997. "Post ADA: Are People with Disabilities Expected to Work?" *Annals of the American Academy of Political and Social Science* 549 (January): 71–83.

Burkhauser, Richard V., and Robert H. Haveman. 1982. *Disability and Work: The Economics of American Policy*. Baltimore: Johns Hopkins University Press.

Ellner, Jack R., and Henry E. Bender. 1980. *Hiring the Handicapped*. New York: Amacom.

Frierson, James G. 1995. *Employer's Guide to the Americans with Disabilities Act*, 2d ed. Washington, D.C.: Bureau of National Affairs.

General Accounting Office. 1996. *People with Disabilities: Federal Programs Could Work Together More Efficiently to Promote Employment*. Washington, D.C.: General Accounting Office.

Growick, Bruce S., and Patrick L. Dunn. 1995. *The Americans with Disabilities Act and Workers' Compensation: Critical Issues and Major Effects*. Horsham, Pa.: LRP Publications.

Lee, Barbara. 1993. "Reasonable Accommodation under the ADA." *Berkeley Journal of Employment and Labor Law* 14: 201.

Martin, Douglas A., and others. 1995. "The ADA and Disability Benefits Policy." *Journal of Disability Policy Studies* 6, no. 2: 1–15.

Mayerson, Arlene. 1991. "Title I–Employment Provisions of the Americans with Disabilities Act." *Temple Law Review* 64, no. 2: 499–520.

Mudrick, Nancy R. 1997. "Employment Discrimination Laws for Disability: Utilization and Outcome." *Annals of the American Academy of Political and Social Science* (January): 53–70.

O'Brien, Ruth. 2001. *Crippled Justice: The History of Modern Disability Policy in the Workplace.* Chicago: University of Chicago Press.

Pimental, Richard, and others. 1993. *The Workers' Compensation-ADA Connection.* Chatsworth, Calif.: Milt Wright and Associates.

Ross, Ruth-Ellen. 1997. *Fifty Years of Progress: An Overview of the President's Committee on Employment of People with Disabilities.* Washington, D.C.: President's Committee on Employment of People with Disabilities.

Tucker, Bonnie. 1991. "The EEOC's Safety Defense Under Title I of the ADA: Valid or Invalid?" *National Disability Law Reporter* 2: 5.

———. 1992. "The Americans with Disabilities Act: Interpreting the Title I Regulations: The Hard Cases." *Cornell Journal of Law and Public Policy* 2, no. 1: 1–24.

Weaver, Carolyn L., ed. 1991. *Disability and Work: Incentives, Rights, and Opportunities.* Washington, D.C.: AEI Press.

Yelin, Edward H. 1992. *Disability and the Displaced Worker.* New Brunswick, N.J.: Rutgers University Press.

Zimmer, Arno B. 1981. *Employing the Handicapped: A Practical Compliance Guide.* New York: Amacom.

HEALTH CARE

Batavia, Andrew I. 1993. "Health Care Reform and People with Disabilities." *Health Affairs* 12, no. 1–2: 40–57.

Brookings Institution. 1995. *Persons with Disabilities: Issues in Health Care Financing and Service Delivery.* Washington, D.C.: Brookings Institution Press.

DeSario, Jack P. 1994. "To Provide Medical Care to Persons with HIV/AIDS: The Americans with Disabilities Act and Refusals." *John Marshall Law Review* 27 (winter): 347.

Feldblum, Chai R. 1991. "Medical Examinations and Inquiries under the Americans with Disabilities Act." *Temple Law Review* 64: 521–49.

Golden, Marilyn. 1991. "Americans with Disabilities Act of 1990: Implications for the Medical Field." *Western Journal of Medicine* 154: 522–24.

Gostin, Lawrence O. 1992. "The Americans with Disabilities Act and the U.S. Health System." *Health Affairs* 11: 248–57.

Grabois, Ellen W., and Margaret A. Nosek. 2001. "The Americans with Disabilities Act and Medical Providers: Ten Years after Passage of the Act." *Policy Studies Journal* 29, no. 4: 682–89.

Grabois, Ellen W., Margaret A. Nosek, and C. D. Rossi. 1999. "The Accessibility of Primary Care Physicians' Offices for People with Disabilities: An Analysis of Compliance with the Americans with Disabilities Act." *Archives of Family Medicine* 8: 44–51.

Handelman, Gwen. 1993. *Health Benefit Plans and the Americans with Disabilities Act.* Horsham, Pa.: LRP Publications.

National Council on Disability. 1993. *Sharing the Risk and Ensuring Independence: A Disability Perspective on Access to Health Insurance and Health-Related Services.* Washington, D.C.: National Council on Disability.

———. 1994. *Making Health Care Reform Work for Americans with Disabilities.* (January 16). Washington, D.C.: National Council on Disability.

Slack, James D. 2001. "The ADA and Reasonable Accommodation: The View from Persons with HIV/AIDS." *Policy Studies Journal* 29, no. 4: 649–53.

Turner, Ronald. 1993. "AIDS, the Americans with Disabilities Act, and Disability-Based Insurance Distinctions." *AIDS and Public Policy Journal* 8, no. 4 (winter): 177–81.

Watson, Sara. 1992. "Reality Ignored: Health Reform and People with Disabilities." *Journal of American Health Policy* 3, no. 2: 49–54.

———. 1993. "An Alliance at Risk: The Disability Movement and Health Care Reform." *The American Prospect* 12 (winter): 60–67.

History

Burgdorf, Marcia P., and Robert Burgdorf, Jr. 1975. "A History of Unequal Treatment." *Santa Clara Lawyer* 35: 855–910.

Covey, Herbert C. 1998. *Social Perceptions of People with Disabilities in History.* Springfield, Ill.: Charles C. Thomas.

Gallagher, Hugh G. 1985. *FDR's Splendid Deception.* New York: Dodd, Mead.

———. 1990. *By Trust Betrayed: Patients, Physicians, and the License to Kill in the Third Reich.* New York: Holt.

Longmore, Paul K. 1987. "Uncovering the Hidden History of People with
    Disabilities." *Reviews in American History* (September): 363.
Scotch, Richard K., and Edward D. Berkowitz. 1990. "One Comprehensive
    System? A Historical Perspective on Federal Disability Policy." *Journal of
    Disability Policy Studies* 1, no. 3 (fall): 1–18.
Scotch, Richard K., and Kay Schriner. 1997. "Disability as Human Variation:
    Implications for Policy." *The Annals of the American Academy of Political and
    Social Science* (January): 148–72.
Treanor, Richard B. 1993. *We Overcame: The Story of Civil Rights for Disabled
    Persons*. Falls Church, Va.: Regal Direct Publishing.
Weicker, Lowell P. Jr. 1991. "Historical Background of the Americans with
    Disabilities Act." *Temple Law Review* 64: 387–92.

Housing

Bazelon Center for Mental Health Law. 1994. *What Does Fair Housing Mean to
    People with Disabilities?* Washington, D.C.: Bazelon Center for Mental
    Healthy Law.
Bull, Ruth. 1998. *Housing Options for Disabled People*. Philadelphia: J. Kingsley.
Goldsmith, Selwyn. 1997. *Designing for the Disabled: The New Paradigm*.
    Boston: Architectural Press.
Preiser, Wolfgang F. E., and Elaine Ostroff, eds. 2001. *Universal Design
    Handbook*. New York: McGraw-Hill.
U.S. Department of Housing and Urban Development. 1997. *Housing
    Opportunities for Persons with Disabilities: Choice, Access, and Communities*.
    Washington, D.C.: Office of Disabilities Policies.

Identity and Culture

Beers, Clifford W. 1908. *A Mind that Found Itself*. New York: Doubleday and
    Company.
Brown, Steven E. 2000. *A Celebration of Diversity: An Annotated Bibliography
    about Disability Culture*. Las Cruces, N.M.: Institute on Disability Culture.
Callahan, John. 1989. *Don't Worry, He Won't Get Far on Foot*. New York: Vintage
    Books.

———. 1992. *Do What He Says! He's Crazy!!!* New York: Quill.

Fries, Kenny. 1997. *Body, Remember: A Memoir.* New York: Plume.

———. 1998. *Staring Back: The Disability Experience from the Inside Out.* New York: Plume.

Gallagher, Hugh Gregory. 1998. *Black Bird Fly Away: Disabled in an Able-Bodied World.* Arlington, Va.: Vandamere Press.

Grandin, Temple. 1995. *Thinking in Pictures and Other Reports from My Life with Autism.* New York: Doubleday and Company.

Hockenberry, John. 1995. *Moving Violations: War Zones, Wheelchairs, and Declarations of Independence.* New York: Hyperion.

Kriegel, Leonard. 1990. *Flying Solo: Reimaging Manhood, Courage and Loss.* Boston: Beacon Press.

Kuusisto, Stephen. 1998. *Planet of the Blind.* New York: Delta.

Mairs, Nancy. 1998. *Waist High in the World: A Life among the Nondisabled.* Boston: Beacon Press.

Murphy, Robert Francis. 2001. *The Body Silent: The Different World of the Disabled.* New York: W. W. Norton.

Robillard, Albert B. 1999. *Meaning of a Disability: The Lived Experience of Paralysis.* Philadelphia: Temple University Press.

Sacks, Oliver W. 1990. *Seeing Voices: A Journey into the World of the Deaf.* Berkeley: University of California Press.

Tuttle, Cheryl G., and Gerald A. Tuttle, eds. 1995. *Challenging Voices: Writings by, for, and about Persons with Learning Disabilities.* Los Angeles: Lowell House.

Wright, Mary Herring. 1999. *Sounds Like Home: Growing Up Black and Deaf in the South.* Washington, D.C.: Gallaudet University Press.

Zola, Irving K. 1982. *Missing Pieces: A Chronicle of Living with a Disability.* Philadelphia: Temple University Press.

LANGUAGE

Longmore, Paul. 1985. "A Note on Language and the Social Identity of Disabled People." *American Behavioral Scientist* 28, no. 3 (January–February): 419–23.

Wilson, James C. 2002. *Embodied Rhetorics: Disability in Language and Culture.* Carbondale: Southern Illinois University Press.

Zola, Irving K. 1988. "The Language of Disability: Problems of Politics and Practice." *Journal of the Disability Advisory Council of Australia* 1, no. 3: 13–21.

LEGAL RIGHTS

Burgdorf, Robert L., Jr. 1980. *The Legal Rights of Handicapped Persons: Cases, Materials, and Text.* Baltimore: Paul H. Brookes.

———. 1997. "'Substantially Limited' Protection from Disibility Discrimination: The Special Treatment Model and Misconstructions of the Definition of Disability." *Villanova Law Review* 42: 107.

DuBow, Sy, Sarah Geer, and Karen Peltz Strauss. 1992. *Legal Rights: The Guide for Deaf and Hard of Hearing People*, 4th ed. Washington, D.C.: Gallaudet University Press.

Frances, Leslie Pickering, and Anita Silvers, eds. 2000. *Americans with Disabilities: Exploring Implications of the Law for Individuals and Institutions.* New York: Routledge.

Gardner, Elaine. 1994. "The Legal Rights of Inmates with Physical Disabilities." *St. Louis University Public Law Review* 14: 175.

Goldman, Charles D. 1987. *Disability Rights Guide: Practical Solutions to Problems Affecting People with Disabilities.* Lincoln, Neb.: Media Publishing.

Parens, Erik, and Adrienne Asch, eds. 2001. *Prenatal Testing and Disability Rights.* Washington, D.C.: Georgetown University Press.

Tucker, Bonnie P., and Bruce A Goldstein. 1992. *Legal Rights of Persons with Disabilities.* Horsham, Pa.: LRP Publications.

MEDIA

Biklen, Douglas. 1986. "Framed: Journalism's Treatment of Disability." *Social Policy* 17, no.1 (winter): 44–51.

Gartner, Alan, and Tom Joe, eds. 1987. *Images of the Disabled, Disabling Images.* New York: Praeger.

Haller, Beth. 1995. "Rethinking Models of Media Representation of Disability." *Disability Studies Quarterly* 15, no. 2 (spring): 35–48.

LaCheen, Cary. 2000. "Achy Breaky Pelvis, Lumber Lung and Juggler's
    Despair: The Portrayal of the Americans with Disability Act on Television
    and Radio." *Berkeley Journal of Employment and Labor Law* 21, no. 1: 223–45.

Nelson, Jack A., ed. 1994. *The Disabled, the Media, and the Information Age.*
    Westport, Conn.: Greenwood Press.

President's Committee on Employment of Persons with Disabilities. 1999. *The
    Disability Messenger: A Guide to Disability Coverage.* Washington, D.C.:
    President's Committee on Employment of Persons with Disabilities.

Shapiro, Joseph. 1994. "Disability Policy and the Media: A Stealth Civil Rights
    Movement Bypasses the Press and Defies Conventional Wisdom." *Policy
    Studies Journal* 22, no. 1 (spring): 123–32.

Wolfe, Kathi. 1996. "Heroes and Holy Innocents: In Portraying Disabled
    People, Hollywood Hasn't Got a Clue." *Utne Reader* (January–February):
    24–26.

Zinn, Harlan. 1995. *Media Stereotypes of Mental Illness, Their Role in Promoting
    Stigma, and Advocacy Efforts to Overcome Such Stereotypes and Stigma.* New
    York: National Stigma Clearinghouse.

Zola, Irving K. 1985. "Depictions of Disability—Metaphor, Message, and
    Medium in the Media: A Research and Political Agenda." *Social Science
    Journal* 22 (1985): 5–17.

Mental Illness

Behrman, Andy. 2002. *Electroboy.* New York: Random House.

Fuller, E., and Judy Miller. 2002. *The Invisible Plague: The Rise of Mental Illness
    from 1750 to the Present Day.* New Brunswick, N.J.: Rutgers University Press.

Grobe, Jeanine, ed. 1995. *Beyond Bedlam: Contemporary Women Psychiatric
    Survivors Speak Out.* Chicago: Third Side Press.

Laden, Vicki A., and Gregory Schwartz. 2000. "Psychiatric Disabilities, the
    ADA, and the New Workplace Violence Account." *Berkeley Journal of
    Employment and Labor Law* 21, no. 1: 246–70.

Neugeboren, Jay. 2001. *New Lives for People Living with Mental Illness.*
    Berkeley: University of California Press.

Porter, Roy. 1989. *A Social History of Madness: The World through the Eyes of the
    Insane.* New York: Dutton.

Stefan, Susan. 2001. *Unequal Rights: Discrimination against People with Mental Disabilities and the Americans with Disabilities Act.* Washington, D.C.: American Psychological Association.

MENTAL RETARDATION

American Association on Mental Retardation. 1996. *Quality of Life.* Washington, D.C.: American Association on Mental Retardation.

Braddock, David. 1986. "From Roosevelt to Reagan: Federal Spending for Mental Retardation and Developmental Disabilities." *American Journal of Mental Deficiency* 90: 479–89.

Dudley, James R. 1997. *Confronting the Stigma in Their Lives.* Springfield, Ill.: C. C. Thomas.

Ferguson, Philip M. 1994. *Abandoned to Their Fate: Social Policy and Practice toward Severely Retarded People in America, 1820–1920.* Philadelphia: Temple University Press.

Perske, Robert. 1991. *Unequal Justice? What Can Happen when Persons with Retardation or Other Developmental Disabilities Encounter the Criminal Justice System.* Nashville, Tenn.: Abingdon Press.

President's Committee on Mental Retardation. 1977. *Mental Retardation: Past and Present.* Washington, D.C.: President's Committee on Mental Retardation.

Smith, J. D. 1985. *Minds Made Feeble: The Myth and Legacy of the Kallikaks.* Rockville, Md.: Aspen Systems.

Taylor, Stephen J. 1996. "Disability Studies and Mental Retardation." *Disability Studies Quarterly* 16, no. 3 (summer): 3–6.

Trent, James W., Jr. 1994. *Inventing the Feeble Mind: A History of Mental Retardation in the United States.* Berkeley: University of California Press.

PERSONAL ASSISTANCE SERVICES

Kennedy, Jae. 1993. "Policy and Program Issues in Providing Personal Assistance Services." *Journal of Rehabilitation* 59, no. 3 (August/September): 17–23.

Litvak, Simi. 1992. "Financing Personal Assistance Services." *Journal of Disability Policy Studies* 3, no. 1: 105.

Marfisi, Carol. 2002. "Personally Speaking: A Critical Reflection of Factors which Blur the Original Vision of Personal Assistance Services." *Disability Studies Quarterly* 22, no. 1. Available at www.cds.hawaii.edu/dsq/issues (accessed March 10, 2002).

Nosek, Margaret A., and Carol A. Howland, 1993. "Personal Assistance Services: The Hub of the Policy Wheel for Community Integration of People with Severe Physical Disabilities." *Policy Studies Journal* 21, no. 4: 789–800.

Pelka, Fred. 1993. "Personal Assistance Services: A Critical Element of Health Care Reform." *Mainstream* 17, no.7 (April): 25–31.

World Institute on Disability. 1990. *The Need for Personal Assistance.* New Brunswick, N.J.: Rutgers University Press.

RELIGION

Betenbaugh, Helen R. 1996. "ADA and the Religious Community: The Moral Case." *Journal of Religion in Disability and Rehabilitation* 2, no. 4: 47–69.

Charleston, James. 1993. "Religion and Disability: A World View." *Disability Rag and Resource*, 14, no. 5 (September/October): 14–16.

Eisland, Nancy L. 1994. *The Disabled God: Toward a Liberatory Theology of Disability.* Nashville, Tenn.: Abingdon Press.

Pietsch, Robert. 1996. "Becoming the Kingdom of God: Building Bridges Between Religion, Secular Society, and Persons with Disabilities." *Journal of Religion in Disability and Rehabilitation* 2, no. 4: 15–25.

Wolfe, Kathi. 1993. "The Bible and Disabilities: From 'Healing' to the 'Burning Bush.'" *Disability Rag and Resources* 14, no. 3 (September–October): 9–10.

SOCIAL SECURITY

Derthick, Martha. 1990. *Agency under Stress: The Social Security Administration in American Government.* Washington, D.C.: Brookings Institution Press.

General Accounting Office. 1996. *Social Security: Disability Programs Lag in Promoting Return to Work.* Testimony before the Special Committee on Aging, U.S. Senate (June 5).

———. 1997. *Social Security: Disability in Promoting Return to Work.* Washington, D.C.: General Accounting Office.

Mezey, Susan G. 1988. *No Longer Disabled: The Federal Courts and the Politics of Social Security Disability.* Westport, Conn.: Greenwood Press.

Quadagno, Jill. 1988. *The Transformation of Old Age Security.* Chicago: University of Chicago Press.

Witte, Edwin E. 1962. *The Development of the Social Security Act.* Madison: University of Wisconsin Press.

SOCIOLOGICAL ASPECTS

Albrecht, Gary L., ed. 1976. *The Sociology of Physical Disability and Rehabilitation.* Pittsburgh: University of Pittsburgh Press.

Barnartt, Sharon N. 1996. "Disability Culture or Disability Consciousness?" *Journal of Disability Policy Studies* 7, no. 2: 1–19.

Barnes, Colin, Geoff Mercer, and Tom Shakespeare. 1999. *Exploring Disability: A Sociological Introduction.* Malden, Mass.: Polity Press.

Barton, Len, ed. 1996. *Disability and Society: Emerging Issues and Insights.* New York: Longman.

Ingstad, Benedicte, and Susan Reynolds Whyte. 1995. *Disability and Culture.* Berkeley: University of California Press.

Oliver, Michael. 1990. *The Politics of Disablement: A Sociological Approach.* New York: St. Martin's Press.

Reinders, Hans S. 2000. *The Future of the Disabled in Liberal Society.* Notre Dame, Ind.: University of Notre Dame Press.

Russell, Marta. 1998. *Beyond Ramps: Disability at the End of the Social Contract.* Monroe, Me.: Common Courage Press.

Smart, Julie. 2001. *Disability, Society, and the Individual.* Gaithersburg, Md.: Aspen Press.

TECHNOLOGY

Alliance for Technology Access. 1996. *Computer Resources for Persons with Disabilities.* Alameda, Calif.: Hunter House Publishers.

Attorney General of the United States. 2000. *Information Technology and Persons with Disabilities: The Current State of Federal Accessibility.* Washington, D.C.: Department of Justice.

Bain, Beverly K., and Dawn Leger. 1997. *Assistive Technology: An Interdisciplinary Approach.* New York: Churchill Livingstone.

Bayha, Betsy. 1998. *The Internet: An Inclusive Magnet for Teaching All Students.* Oakland, Calif.: World Institute on Disability.

Bowe, Frank G. 1994. "Access to the Information Age: Fundamental Decisions in Telecommunications Policy." *Policy Studies Journal* 21, no. 4: 765–74.

Cunningham, Carmela, and Norman Coombs. 1997. *Information Access and Adaptive Technology.* Phoenix: American Council on Education and Oryx Press.

Espinola, Olga. 1999. *Captured by the Net.* Boston: National Braille Press.

Forsythe, Chris, Eric Grose, and Julie Ratner, eds. 1998. *Human Factors and Web Development.* Mahwah, N.J.: Lawrence Erlbaum Associates.

Gray, David B., Louis A. Quatrano, and Morton L. Lieberman, eds. 1998. *Designing and Using Assistive Technology: The Human Perspective.* Baltimore: Paul H. Brookes.

King, Thomas W. 1999. *Assistive Technology: Essential Human Factors.* Boston: Allyn & Bacon.

Lane, Joseph P. 1997. "Technology Evaluation and Transfer in the Assistive Technology Marketplace: Terms, Process, and Roles." *Technology and Disability* 7 (June): 5–24.

Mates, Barbara, Doug Wakefield, and Judith Dixon. 2001. *Adaptive Technology for the Internet: Making Electronic Resources Accessible to All.* Chicago: American Library Association.

National Council on Disability. 1996. *Access to the Information Superhighway and Emerging Information Technologies by People with Disabilities.* Washington, D.C.: National Council on Disability.

Senge, Jeffrey C. 1997. "How Technology Has Improved My Access to Information." *Technology and Disability* 6 (May): 191–98.

TRANSPORTATION

Clark, Timothy B. 1980. "Regulation Gone Amok: How Many Billions for Wheelchair Transit?" *Regulation* 4 (March/April): 47–52.

Fix, Michael, Carol Everett, and Ronald Kirby. 1985. *Providing Transportation to the Disabled: Local Responses to Evolving Federal Policies.* Washington, D.C.: Urban Institute.

General Accounting Office. 1994. *Americans with Disabilities Act: Challenges Faced by Transit Agencies in Complying with the Act's Requirements.* Washington, D.C.: U.S. General Accounting Office.

Katzmann, Robert A. 1986. *Institutional Disability: The Saga of Transportation Policy for the Disabled.* Washington, D.C.: Brookings Institution Press.

Muller, Henrik. 1977. *Airlines and Disabled Travelers.* Stockholm: International Society for Rehabilitation of the Disabled.

Pfeiffer, David. 1990. "Public Transit Access for Disabled Persons in the United States." *Disability, Handicap, and Society* 5: 153–66.

Scherer, Marcia J. 2000. *Living in the State of Stuck: How Assistive Technology Impacts the Lives of People with Disabilities.*, 3d ed. Cambridge, Mass.: Brookline Books.

U.S. Department of Transportation. 1991. *Preliminary Regulatory Impact Analysis of Transportation Accessibility Requirements for the Americans with Disabilities Act.* Washington, D.C.: U.S. Department of Transportation.

U.S. Office of Technology Assessment. 1993. *Access to Over-the-Road Buses for Persons with Disabilities.* Washington, D.C.: U.S. Office of Technology Assessment.

Winter, Michael A., and Fred Laurence Williams. 2001. "Transit Access for Americans." *Policy Studies Journal* 29, no. 4: 674–81.

VOTING

Armstrong, Barbara. 1976. "The Mentally Disabled and the Right to Vote." *Hospital and Community Psychiatry* 27 (August): 577–82.

Federal Election Commission. 1996. *Ensuring the Accessibility of the Election Process.* Washington, D.C.: Federal Election Commission.

Note. 1979. "Mental Disability and the Right To Vote." *Yale Law Journal* 88: 1644–64.

Schriner, Kay, and Andrew Batavia. 2001. "The ADA: Does It Secure the Fundamental Right to Vote?" *Policy Studies Journal* 29, no. 4: 663–73.

Schriner, Kay, Lisa O. Ochs, and Todd G. Shields. 1997. "The Last Suffrage Movement: Voting Rights for Persons with Cognitive and Emotional Disabilities." *Publius* 27, no. 3 (summer): 75–96.

WOMEN AND DISABILITIES

Asch, Adrienne, and Michelle Fine, eds. 1988. *Women with Disabilities: Essays in Psychology, Culture, and Politics.* Philadelphia: Temple University Press.

Driedger, Diane, ed. 1996. *Across Borders: Women with Disabilities Working Together.* Charlottetown, Prince Edward Is.: Gynergy Books.

Frank, Gelya. 2000. *Venus on Wheels: Two Decades of Dialogue on Disability, Biography, and Being Female in America.* Berkeley: University of California Press.

Hillyer, Barbara. 1993. *Feminism and Disability.* Norman: University of Oklahoma Press.

Morris, Jenny, ed. 1996. *Encounters with Strangers: Femininity and Disability.* London: Women's Press.

Nosek, Margaret A., and others. 1997. *National Study of Women with Physical Disabilities: Final Report.* Houston: Center for Research on Women with Disabilities.

Resources for Rehabilitation. 2000. *A Woman's Guide to Coping with Disability.* Lexington, Mass.: Resources for Rehabilitation.

Rousso, Harilyn. 1993. *Disabled, Female, and Proud!* Westport, Conn.: Bergin and Garvey.

Traustadottir, Rannveig. 1990. *Women with Disabilities: Issues, Resources, Connections.* Syracuse, N.Y.: Center on Human Policy.

U.S. Department of Labor. 1992. *Women with Work Disabilities.* Washington, D.C.: U.S. Department of Labor.

APPENDIX B

Selected Disability Periodicals and Media

Note: Most of these publications are available online only. Mailing addresses are available as indicated.

Abilities. Canadian Abilities Foundation, 489 College Street, Suite 501, Toronto ON M6G 1A5. (416) 923-1885. www.enablelink.org

ABILITY Magazine. 1001 West 17th Street, Costa Mesa, CA 92627. (949) 854-8700. www.abilitymagazine.com

Accent on Living Magazine. P.O. Box 700, Bloomington, IL 61702-0700. (800) 787-8444

AccessWorld. AFB Press. (800) 232-3044. www.afb.org

American Council of the Blind Radio. www.acbradio.org

AnAurora Magazine for Women. www.anAurora.co.uk

Braille Forum. www.acb.org/magazine

Braille Monitor. 1800 Johnson Street, Baltimore, MD 20230. (410) 659-9314 www.nfb.org/bralmons

Chronic Fatigue Syndrome Electronic Newsletter. www.cfs-news.org/cfs-news

Closing the Gap. Closing the Gap, P.O. Box 68, Henderson, MN 56044. (507) 248-3294. www.closingthegap.com

Council for Exceptional Children On-Line. 1110 North Glebe Road, Suite 300, Arlington, VA 22201-5704. (888) 232-7733. www.cec.sped.org

Deaf-Blind Perspectives. Teaching Research Division, Western Oregon State College, 345 N. Monmouth Avenue, Monmouth, OR 97344. (503) 838-8598

Dialogue Magazine. PO Box 5181, Salem, OR 97304-0181. (800) 860-4224. www.blindskills.com

Disability and Society. Taylor and Francis, 11 New Fetter Lane, London EC4P 4EE, England

Disability International. 101-7 Evergreen Place, Winnipeg, Manitoba, R3L 2T3 Canada. (204) 287-8010

Disability Resources Monthly. www.disabilityresources.org

Disabilities Studies Online Magazine. www.disabilitystudies.com

Disability Studies Quarterly. www.cds.hawaii.edu/DSQ

Disability Times. 84 Claverton Street, London SW1V 3AX, England. 020 7233–7970. www.disabilitytimes.com

Disability World. www.disabilityworld.org

Eastern Paralyzed Veterans Association Action. www.epva.org/EPVA_Action

Enabled Online. www.enabledonline.com

Hearing Health Magazine. P.O. Drawer V, Ingleside, TX 78362. (512) 776-7240 V/TTY

iCAN Online. www.icanonline.net

Inclusion Daily Express. P.O. Box 68, Spangle, WA 99031. (888) 551-8280. www.InclusionDaily.com

Journal of Disability Policy Studies. Pro-ed, 8700 Shoal Creek Blvd., Austin, TX 78757-6897. (512) 451-3246

Justice For All E-Network. www.jfanow.org

Little People of America Online. Box 745, Lubbock, TX 79408. (888) 572-2001. www.lpaonline.org

Mainstream Magazine Online. www.mainstream-mag.com

Mouth. P.O. Box 558, Topeka, KS 66601. www.mouthmag.com

National Alliance for the Mentally Ill E-News. www.nami.org/update

National Organization on Disability E-Newsletter. www.nod.org

New Mobility Magazine. P.O. Box 220, Horsham, PA 19044. (215) 675-9133. www.newmobility.com

On a Roll Radio. www.onarollradio.com

Ragged Edge Magazine. P.O. Box 145, Louisville, KY 40201. www.raggededgemagazine.com

Reach Out Magazine. 3090 Sheridan Street, PMB #207, Hollywood, FL 33021-3730. (954) 985-0319. www.reachoutmag.com

Technology and Disability. IOS Press, Inc., 5795-G Burke Center Parkway, Burke, VA 22015.

Volta Review; Volta Voices. 3417 Volta Place NW, Washington, DC 20007. (202) 337-5220. www.agbell.org

WE Magazine. 130 William Street, New York, NY 10038. (212) 375-6266. www.wemedia.com

APPENDIX C

Annotated Guide to Nongovernmental Disability Organizations

Adaptive Environments Center/www.adaptenv.org
374 Congress Street, Suite 301
Boston, MA 02210
(617) 695-1225 voice/TDD
Promotes accessibility through design consultation, education programs, publications, and ADA technical assistance.

Alexander Graham Bell Association for the Deaf/www.agbell.org
3417 Volta Place NW
Washington, DC 20007
(202) 337-5220
Gathers and disseminates information on hearing loss and advocates for the rights of children and adults who are hard of hearing or deaf.

Alliance for Technology Access/www.ataccess.org
2175 East Francisco Boulevard, Suite L
San Rafael, CA 94901
(415) 455-4575
Network of community-based resource centers, developers, and vendors to provide information and support for accessible technology.

American Association of People with Disabilities/www.aapd-dc.org
1819 H Street NW, Suite 330

Washington, DC 20006

(800) 840-8844

Nonprofit, nonpartisan cross-disability organization that promotes unity and
leadership.

American Association of the Deaf-Blind/www.tr.wou.edu/dblink/aadb.htm

814 Thayer Avenue, Room 302

Silver Spring, MD 20910-4500

(800) 735-2258

Promotes better opportunities and services for deaf-blind people.

American Association on Mental Retardation/www.aamr.org

444 North Capitol Street NW, Suite 846

Washington, DC 20001-1512

(800) 424-3688

Works to increase awareness about mental retardation and related conditions.

American Bar Association Commission on Mental and Physical Disability Law

www.abanet.org/disability

740 15th Street NW

Washington, DC 20005

(202) 662-1570

Provides legal aid and advocacy; publishes law journal, citation database, and
registry of lawyers specializing in disability law.

American Council of the Blind/www.acb.org

1155 15th Street NW, Suite 1004

Washington, DC 20005

(800) 424-8666

Seeks to improve the well-being of persons who are blind by serving as a representative national organization.

American Diabetes Foundation/www.diabetes.org

1701 N. Beauregard Street

Alexandria, VA 22311

(800) 342-2383

Provides information, support, and advocacy for persons with diabetes.

American Disabled for Attendant Programs Today (ADAPT)/www.adapt.org
201 S. Cherokee
Denver, CO 80223
(303) 733-9324
Advocacy group seeking support for personal attendant programs for people
    with disabilities.

American Foundation for the Blind/www.afb.org
11 Penn Plaza, Suite 300
New York, NY 10001
(800) 232-5463
Founded in 1912 to serve as a resource for persons who are blind and visually
    impaired.

American Institute of Architects/www.aiaonline.com
1735 New York Avenue NW
Washington, D.C. 20006
(202) 626-7300
Professional society of architects and source of accessible design resources.

American Society for Deaf Children/www.deafchildren.org
PO Box 3355
Gettysburg, PA 17325
(717) 334-7922 V/TTY
Nonprofit parent-helping organization promoting a positive attitude toward
    signing and deaf culture.

Arthritis Foundation/www.arthritis.org
PO Box 7669
Atlanta, GA 30357-0669
(800) 283-7800
Organization works to improve lives through leadership in the prevention, con-
    trol, and cure of arthritis-related diseases.

Association for Persons with Severe Handicaps (see TASH)

Association of Programs for Rural Independent Living
  (APRIL)/www.april.umt.edu
5903 Powdermill Road
Kent, OH 44240
(330) 678-7648
National clearinghouse for centers of independent living and others working in
  rural areas.

Association on Higher Education and Disability (AHEAD)/www.ahead.org
University of Massachusetts, Boston
100 Morrissey Boulevard
Boston, MA 02125-3393
(617) 287-3880
Provides policy guidance on accessibility, accommodations, and information
  for postsecondary educators and administrators.

Attention Deficit Information Network/www.addinfonetwork.com
58 Prince Street
Needham, MA 02492
(781) 455-9895
Volunteer organization to provide resources, training, and conferences on
  ADD.

Autism Society of America/www.autism-society.org
7910 Woodmont Avenue, Suite 300
Bethesda, MD 20814-3067
(800) 328-8476
Promotes lifelong access and opportunities for people along the autism
  spectrum.

Bazelon Center for Mental Health Law/www.bazelon.org
1101 15th Street NW, Suite 1212
Washington, DC 20005-5002
(202) 223-0409
Nonprofit legal advocacy organization for people with mental illness and mental retardation.

Center for Universal Design/www.design.ncsc.edu/cud
School of Design, North Carolina State University
Box 8613
Raleigh, NC 27695-8613
(800) 647-6777
Provides technical assistance, training, and publications on accessible design.

Cochlear Implant Association/www.cici.org
5335 Wisconsin Avenue NW, Suite 440
Washington, DC 20015-2052
(202) 895-2781 V/TTY
Provides information and support to cochlear implant users and their families,
    professionals, and the general public and advocates for deaf people.

Consortium for Citizens with Disabilities/www.c-c-d.org
1730 K Street NW, Suite 1212
Washington, DC 20006
(202) 785-3388
Coalition of more than 100 national disability organizations to advocate on
    behalf of persons with disabilities.

Council for Disability Rights/www.disabilityrights.org
205 West Randolph, Suite 1645
Chicago, IL 60606
(312) 444-9484
Provides information, advocacy, education, counseling, and job training.

Council for Exceptional Children/www.cec.sped.org
1110 North Glebe Road, Suite 300
Arlington, VA 22201-5704
(888) 232-7733
Advocates on behalf of children and provides resources and support.

Disability Resources, Inc./www.disabilityresources.org
Online nonprofit organization that monitors and disseminates information
    about disabilities.

Disability Rights Advocates/www.dralegal.org

449 15th Street, Suite 303

Oakland, CA 94612-2821

(510) 451-8644

Legal advocacy program litigating on behalf of persons with disabilities.

Disability Rights Education and Defense Fund, Inc./www.dredf.org

2212 Sixth Street

Berkeley, CA 94710

(510) 644-2555 V/TTY

National law and policy center protecting and advocating civil rights of persons
with disabilities.

Disabled Peoples International/www.dpi.org

101-7 Evergreen Place

Winnipeg, Manitoba

Canada R3L 2T3

(204) 287-8010

International organization that works to develop partnerships and linkages with
government, business, and the academic world to achieve full participation
and equality.

Eastern Paralyzed Veterans Association/www.epva.org

75-20 Astoria Boulevard

Jackson Heights, NY 11370-1177

(718) 803-EPVA

Major chapter of Paralyzed Veterans of America; sponsor of wide range of programs and wheelchair sports activities.

Epilepsy Foundation/www.efa.org

4351 Garden City Drive

Landover, MD 20785-7223

(800) 332-1000

Foundation works to serve all persons with seizure disorders through research,
education, advocacy, and service.

International Dyslexia Association/www.interdys.org
8600 La Salle Road
382 Chester Building
Baltimore, MD 21286-2044
(410) 296-0232
Assists persons with dyslexia and other learning disorders, providing information and education.

Job Accommodation Network (JAN)/www.janweb.icdi.wvu.edu
PO Box 6080
Morgantown, WV 26506-6080
(800) 526-7234 (V/TTY)
Toll-free consulting service that provides information about job accommoda-
tions and employment of people with disabilities under auspices of U.S.
Department of Labor.

Justice for All/www.jfanow.org
E-mail network to disseminate information on actions in Congress affecting
persons with disabilities.

League for the Hard of Hearing/www.lhh.org
71 West 23rd Street
New York, NY 10010-4162
(917) 305-7700
Oldest hearing rehabilitation agency in the United States, with a goal of
improving the quality of life for people with all degrees of hearing loss.

Learning Disabilities Association of America/www.ldanatl.org
4156 Library Road
Pittsburgh, PA 15234-1349
(412) 341-1515
Identifies the causes of learning disabilities, ensures effective identification and
diagnosis of individuals who are learning disabled, and promotes the rights
of persons with learning disabilities.

Leukemia and Lymphoma Society of America/www.leukemia.org
1311 Mamaroneck Avenue
White Plains, NY 10605
(914) 949-5213
Fights blood-related cancers and attempts to improve the quality of life for
patients and their families.

Little People of America/www.lpaonline.org
PO Box 65030
Lubbock, TX 79464-5030
(888) LPA-2001
Organization for people of short stature and their families.

Lupus Foundation of America/www.lupus.org
1300 Piccard Drive, Suite 200
Rockville, MD 20850-4303
(301) 670-9292
Organization's goal is to educate and support people affected by lupus and to
find a cure.

MadNation/www.madnation.cc
154 Woodborough Terrace SW
Calgary, AB T2W 5B5 Canada
(403) 281-6265
Canadian-based group working for justice and human rights in mental health,
focusing on involuntary treatment worldwide.

Mainstream, Inc./www.mainstreaminc.org
6930 Carroll Avenue, Suite 240
Takoma Park, MD 20912
Nonprofit organization that develops cost-effective solutions to place people
with disabilities in the workplace.

Mental Disability Rights International/www.mdri.org
1156 15th Street NW, Suite 1001

Washington, DC 20005

(202) 296-0800

Advocates on behalf of individuals with psychiatric illnesses in a joint program
with Bazelon Center.

Mobility International USA/www.mdausa.org

PO Box 10767

Eugene, OR 97440

(541) 343-1284 V/TTY

Non-profit organization providing information on travel and accessible desti-
nations.

Muscular Dystrophy Association/www.mdusa.org

3300 East Sunrise Drive

Tucson, AZ 85718

(800) 572-1717

Promotes research and raises funds for services for persons with neuromuscular
diseases.

National Alliance for the Mentally Ill/www.nami.org

2107 Wilson Boulevard, Suite 300

Arlington, VA 22201

(703) 524-7600

Founded in 1979 as a grassroots self-help, support, and advocacy group to seek
equitable services for people with severe mental illnesses.

National Association for the Visually Handicapped/www.navh.org

22 West 21st Street

New York, NY 10010

(212) 889-3141

Information and referral; direct services, including large-print materials; and
advocacy for persons who are partially sighted.

National Association of the Deaf/www.nad.org

814 Thayer Avenue

Silver Spring, MD 20910-4500

(301) 587-1788

Established in 1880 to safeguard accessibility and civil rights of deaf and hard of
hearing people; also operates NAD Law Center.

National Association of Homebuilders Research Center/www.nahb.com

400 Prince George's Boulevard

Upper Marlboro, MD 20772-8731

(301) 249-4000

Research arm of home-building industry that provides information on housing
accessibility and accessible building products.

National Association of Protection and Advocacy Systems/
www.protectionandadvocacy.com

900 Second Street NE, Suite 211

Washington, DC 20002

(202) 408-9514

Association of federally mandated programs that protect the rights of persons
with disabilities through client assistance programs.

National Center for Dissemination of Disability Research/www.ncddr.org

Southwest Educational Development Laboratory

211 East 7th Street, Room 400

Austin, TX 78701-3281

(800) 266-1832

Disseminates outcomes of disability research, promotes demonstration activities, and provides technical assistance.

National Council on Independent Living/www.ncil.org

1916 Wilson Boulevard, Suite 209

Arlington, VA 22201

(703) 525-3406 V/TTD

Membership organization to advance independent living philosophy and advocate for human rights and services for people with disabilities.

National Disability Party/www.disabilityparty.com
Political organization established in 2000 seeking equal rights and access for all
   persons.

National Down Syndrome Society/www.ndss.org
666 Broadway
New York, NY 10012
(212) 460-9330
Established to ensure that all people with Down syndrome have an opportunity
   to achieve their full potential in community life.

National Easter Seals Society/www.easter-seals.org
230 West Monroe Street, Suite 1800
Chicago, IL 60606
(312) 726-6200
(312) 726-4258 TDY
(800) 221-6827
Umbrella organization founded in 1919 to provide advocacy, research, and education for disabled persons.

National Federation of the Blind/www.nfb.org
1800 Johnson Street
Baltimore, MD 21230
(410) 659-9314
Largest organization of blind persons in America, providing information, support, and advocacy.

National Hemophilia Foundation/www.hemophilia.org
116 West 32nd Street, 11th Floor
New York, NY 10001
(212) 328-3700
Works to prevent or reduce complications of hemophilia.

National Mental Health Association/www.nmha.org
2001 N. Beauregard Street, 12th floor

Alexandria, VA 22311

(703) 684-7722

Works to improve the mental health of all Americans.

National Multiple Sclerosis Society/www.nmss.org

733 Third Avenue

New York, NY 10017

(800) 344-4867

Organizes and supports chapters throughout the United States and serves as
information source.

National Organization on Disability/www.nod.org

910 16th Street, NW, Suite 600

Washington, DC 20006

(202) 293-5960

Serves as coordinating body for disability rights advocacy, information, and
programs.

National Osteoporosis Foundation/www.nof.org

1232 22nd Street, NW

Washington, DC 20037-1292

(202) 223-2226

Provides resources, information, and online support to prevent or reduce the
impact of osteoporosis.

National Spinal Cord Injury Association/www.spinalcord.org

6701 Democracy Boulevard, Suite 300-9

Bethesda, MD 20817

(301) 588-6959

Provides information and advocacy for persons with spinal cord injuries.

Not Dead Yet/www.acils.com/notdeadyet

7521 Madison Street

Forest Park, IL 60130

(708) 209-1500

National organization opposing assisted suicide.

Paralyzed Veterans of America/www.pva.org
801 18th Street NW
Washington, DC 20006-3317
(800) 424-8200
National organization of veterans with spinal cord diseases and injuries that
cause paralysis.

Parkinson's Disease Foundation/www.pdf.org
710 West 168th Street
New York, NY 10032-9982
(800) 457-6676
Provides information, support, and legislative advocacy.

Rehabilitation International/www.rehab-international.org
25 East 21st Street
New York, NY 10010
(212) 420-1500
Federation of organizations working for prevention of disability and rehabilitation of persons with disabilities.

Self Help for Hard of Hearing People (SHHH)/www.shhh.org
7910 Woodmont Avenue, Suite 1200
Bethesda, MD 20814
(301) 657-2249
Promotes awareness and information about hearing loss, communication, assistive devices, and alternative communication skills.

Society for Disability Studies/www.uic.edu/orgs/sds
Department of Disability and Human Development
University of Illinois, Chicago
MC 626
1640 West Roosevelt Road, #236
Chicago, IL 60608-6904
(312) 996-4664 V/TTY
Professional association that promotes and disseminates research on various
issues involving persons with disabilities.

Spina Bifida Association of America/www.sbaa.org

4590 MacArthur Boulevard NW, Suite 250

Washington, DC 20007-4226

(800) 621-3141

Group's mission is to promote prevention of spina bifida and enhance the lives
of all affected.

TASH/www.tash.org

29 West Susquehanna Avenue, Suite 210

Baltimore, MD 21204

(410) 828-8274

International association of persons with disabilities fighting for inclusion in all
aspects of society.

United Cerebral Palsy Association/www.ucpa.org

1660 L Street NW, Suite 700

Washington, DC 20036

(202) 776-0406

(202) 973-7197

Now UCP National, the organization provides resources and information on
cerebral palsy.

Very Special Arts/www.vsarts.org

1300 Connecticut Avenue NW, Suite 700

Washington, DC 20036

(800) 933-8721

(202) 737-0645 TTY

International nonprofit organization dedicated to promoting the creative power
in persons with disabilities.

Western Law Center for Disability Rights/www.wlcdr.everybody.org

919 Albany Street

Los Angeles, CA 90015-1211

(213) 736-1031

Provides legal-related services and promotes disability rights.

World Institute on Disability/www.wid.org
510 16th Street, Suite 100
Oakland, CA 94612
(510) 763-4100
(510) 208-9496 TTY
Nonprofit public policy center carrying out research on disability issues.

APPENDIX D

Chronology of Important Events in the History and Development of American Disability Policy

1812 • School for Blind opens in Baltimore

1817 • Connecticut Asylum for the Education and Instruction of Deaf and Dumb Persons opens in Hartford, Connecticut

1822 • American School for the Deaf adds vocational training to its curriculum

1832 • Perkins School for the Blind in Boston admits its first students

1848 • First residential school for persons with mental retardation opens in Boston

1854 • President Franklin Pierce vetoes bill to provide federal funding for separate facilities for physically and mentally disabled persons, saying it was not a federal responsibility

1861 • Civil War/Union Army amputations estimated at 30,000, creating tremendous need for prosthetic devices and rehabilitation

1869 • First patent for a wheelchair registered with U.S. Patent Office

1911 • Congress authorizes appointment of federal commission to investigate liability of employers for financial compensation to disabled workers

1920 • Fess-Smith Civilian Vocational Rehabilitation Act provides federal assistance to states for services for disabled persons

1921 • Veterans Bureau established to deal with needs of disabled World War I veterans

1927 • U.S. Supreme Court rules in favor of forced sterilization of disabled woman

1929	• First guide dog school for blind persons opens

1929   • First guide dog school for blind persons opens

1932   • Congress mandates Disabled American Veterans to represent their members in dealings with the federal government

1935   • League for the Physically Handicapped protests discrimination by the federal Works Progress Administration and other federal programs
         • Congress passes Social Security Act to provide assistance for blind individuals and disabled children

1938   • Euthanasia Society of America formed, calls for killing defective children by age five

1940   • American Federation of the Physically Handicapped becomes first cross-disability, national political organization in the United States

1945   • President Harry Truman proclaims the first National Employ the Handicapped Week

1947   • President's Committee on Employment of the Handicapped founded

1950   • State programs for aid to persons who are permanently and totally disabled established by Social Security Act Amendments, becoming prototype for future federal legislation
         • University of Illinois sets up first program to help disabled veterans of World War II

1952   • President's Committee on National Employ the Handicapped Week becomes President's Committee on Employment of the Physically Handicapped, a permanent organization reporting to the president and Congress

1954   • Social Security Act Amendments protect benefits of workers who leave workforce because of a disability

1955   • Congress establishes Joint Commission on Mental Illness and Health

1956   • Social Security Amendments extend benefits to dependents of disabled workers

1960   • Elimination of age threshold (age 50) for disabled workers by Social Security Act Amendments

1961   • President Kennedy appoints members to new President's Panel on Mental Retardation
         • American National Standards Institute publishes specifications for accessible buildings, the basis for all subsequent architectural access codes

1963 • Passage of Mental Retardation Facilities and Community Mental Health Centers Construction Act

1964 • Enactment of Civil Rights Act becomes catalyst for activism and eventually serves as a model for disability rights legislation
• Robert Weitbrecht invents telecommunications device for the deaf (TDD)

1965 • Congress establishes Medicare and Medicaid programs to subsidize health care to disabled and elderly persons
• Passage of Vocational Rehabilitation Amendments to authorize construction of rehabilitation centers and create National Commission on Architectural Barriers to Rehabilitation of the Handicapped
• *Christmas in Purgatory* exposes mistreatment of residents of institutions in New York after tour by Senator Robert Kennedy

1966 • President Lyndon Johnson establishes President's Committee on Mental Retardation
• Actor Jerry Lewis takes over as host of Muscular Dystrophy Association Labor Day telethon
• Cued speech invented for use by deaf persons

1967 • Rolling Quads group forms at University of California Berkeley
1968 • Passage of Architectural Barriers Act, mandating that all federally constructed buildings be physically accessible

1969 • White House conference urges "normalization" of people with developmental disabilities

1970 • Rolling Quads group becomes Disabled Students' Program at Berkeley
• Passage of Developmental Disabilities Services and Facilities Construction Amendments, defining developmental disabilities and authorizing services
• Judy Heumann denied license to teach in New York City schools because of her quadriplegia, files successful lawsuit, and founds Disabled in Action

1971 • Center for Independent Living established in Berkeley, California, to provide community living and services for disabled persons
• First legal advocacy program for persons with disabilities established at University of Notre Dame

1972   • Media coverage of conditions at New York's Willowbrook State School exposes inhumane treatment of persons with developmental disabilities, serving as basis for movement toward community-based living centers

• Center for Independent Living incorporated in Berkeley, California

• Disabled in Action leads protests against President Richard Nixon's veto of spending bill to fund disability programs

1973   • Passage of Rehabilitation Act, which prohibits discrimination against persons with disabilities and legitimizes disability rights movement

• Washington, D.C., issues first handicapped parking placards

• Children's Defense Fund study reveals 750,000 disabled children not in schools

1974   • Ron Mace founds Barrier Free Environments to advocate that all buildings and products be accessible

1975   • Passage of Developmentally Disabled Assistance and Bill of Rights Act, including funding to serve persons in institutions

• Passage of Education for All Handicapped Children Act, establishing right to public school education in integrated setting

• California Governor Jerry Brown appoints activist Ed Roberts as head of state's Department of Rehabilitation

1976   • Higher Education Act Amendments establish services for students with disabilities at colleges

1977   • Disabled activists take over San Francisco offices of U.S. Department of Health, Education, and Welfare in longest sit-in at a federal building in U.S. history

• Passage of Education of the Handicapped Amendments

• 1973 Rehabilitation Act Section 504 regulations issued

• First White House Conference on Handicapped Individuals held to recommend changes in federal disability policies

1978   • Passage of the Rehabilitation and Developmental Disabilities Amendments

• ADAPT holds first protest in Denver, blocking intersections and demanding that wheelchair lifts be added to buses

1979
- Department of Health, Education, and Welfare split into two cabinet-level departments: Department of Health and Human Services and Department of Education
- Disability Rights Education and Defense Fund founded in Berkeley, California, becoming major litigator for persons with disabilities

1980
- Thousands of persons with disabilities lose benefits under provisions of Social Security Act Amendments
- Passage of Civil Rights of Institutionalized Persons Act, allowing Department of Justice to file suit on behalf of institutionalized residents

1981
- Activist Evan Kemp, Jr. writes attack on Muscular Dystrophy Association telethon for *New York Times*

1983
- Disabled protesters disrupt American Public Transit Association convention in Denver, Colorado, focusing attention on disabled access to public transportation
- Job Accommodation Network (JAN) established by President's Committee on Employment of the Handicapped to facilitate disabled employment opportunities
- Elizabeth Bouvia asks hospital to administer painkillers while she starves herself to death because of severe cerebral palsy; hospital refuses

1984
- National Council of the Handicapped becomes independent federal agency
- Enactment of Voting Accessibility for the Elderly and Handicapped Act

1985
- Ethicists propose killing of children with severe disabilities in book, *Should the Baby Live?*

1986
- Passage of Protection and Advocacy for Mentally Ill Individuals Act
- Passage of Education of the Handicapped Act Amendments
- Air Carrier Access Act prohibits airlines from refusing to serve disabled passengers
- Actress Marlee Matlin wins Oscar for portrayal of deaf student in movie, *Children of a Lesser God*
- Founding of Society for Disability Studies to unite academicians and researchers

1988   • "Deaf President Now!" protest at Gallaudet University in
              Washington, D.C.
              • Passage of Technology-Related Assistance for Individuals with
              Disabilities Act to promote access to assistive technology
              • Fair Housing Act Amendments enacted to provide protection
              against housing discrimination on the basis of disability
              • Original version of Americans with Disabilities Act (ADA)
              drafted and introduced into Congress
              • National Council on the Handicapped renamed National
              Council on Disability
              • Protestors from National Stuttering Project picket movie theaters
              showing *A Fish Called Wanda*

1989   • Reintroduction of ADA in Congress
              • President's Committee on Employment of the Handicapped
              renamed President's Committee on Employment of People with
              Disabilities
              • *Rain Man* wins Academy Award as best movie; depicts life of
              autistic man
              • Syracuse professor Douglas Biklen visits Australia to see demon-
              stration of facilitated communication (in which a person trained in
              the technique supports or applies mild restraint to the arm of a per-
              son with a disability, allowing the use of a letterboard, pictures, or
              keyboard)
              • Michigan judge allows quadriplegic on respirator to refuse med-
              ical treatment and die with assistance from hospice physician

1990   • Television Decoder Circuitry Act requires closed-caption decoders
              on all televisions thirteen inches and larger
              • Wheels of Justice protest in Washington, D.C., to support
              passage of ADA
              • Jack Kevorkian performs first assisted suicide with "mercy machine"

1991   • Passage of Protection and Advocacy for Mentally Ill Individuals
              Act Amendments
              • International Special Olympics Games in Minneapolis becomes
              biggest sporting event in the world
              • Association of Retarded Citizens changes its name to The ARC to
              reflect demands that the organization not use the term "retarded"

• National Right to Life Committee chooses paraplegic as president to emphasize its opposition to abortion of disabled fetuses
• Loma Linda University ethicist suggests heart transplant from mentally handicapped child to save the life of a healthy baboon or chimpanzee

1992 • Rehabilitation Act of 1973 amended

1995 • Actor Christopher Reeve injures spinal cord in horseback riding incident

1996 • Telecommunications Act enacted to provide equal access to telecommunications for people with disabilities

1997 • Passage of the Individuals with Disabilities Education Act

1998 • President Bill Clinton creates Presidential Task Force on Employment of Adults with Disabilities
• U.S. Appeals Court reaffirms ruling to require dentist to treat patient with AIDS virus
• Enactment of Crime Victims with Disabilities Awareness Act
• Federal agencies ordered to conduct studies to improve access to federal outdoor recreational areas
• Assistive Technology Act of 1998 signed into law
• ADAPT activists occupy Democratic and Republican national headquarters in Washington, D.C., demanding change in institutionally based long-term service system
• American Association of People with Disabilities holds "Show Your Power" events

1999 • U.S. Supreme Court issues ruling in *Olmstead* case on right to receive care in most integrated setting
• Access Board approves proposal for new ADA Accessibility Guidelines
• U.S. Supreme Court rules on definition of disability in several cases
• Equal Employment Opportunity Commission (EEOC) releases policy guidance on reasonable accommodation and undue hardship and duties for employers
• Actor Michael J. Fox testifies before Congress on behalf of research funding for Parkinson's disease
• American Paralysis Association merges with Christopher Reeve Foundation

• Dr. Jack Kevorkian sentenced to prison in Michigan for physician-assisted suicide

2000
• Standards for Electronic and Information Technology issued by Access Board

• Tenth anniversary of signing of ADA, celebrations nationwide

• National Council on Disability releases report on ten years of enforcement of ADA

• Thousands of disabled voters claim they could not find accessible polling places or assistance during presidential election

• Court of Appeals reverses conviction of Kelly Dillery after arrest in Sandusky, Ohio

2001
• President Bill Clinton unveils statue of Franklin D. Roosevelt seated in wheelchair at FDR Memorial

• U.S. Supreme Court rules on discrimination and ADA Title II

• President George W. Bush creates Office of Disability Employment Policy

• Section 508 of Rehabilitation Act Amendments of 1998 becomes law

• U.S. Supreme Court rules disabled golfer Casey Martin can use golf cart

• President George W. Bush announces New Freedom Initiative

• Michigan Court of Appeals denies request by Dr. Jack Kevorkian for a new trial

• Bush administration releases report on *Federal Agencies' Actions to Eliminate Barriers and Promote Community Integration*

2002
• U.S. Supreme Court restricts application of ADA to employees with permanent or long-term disabilities

• States begin implementation of Ticket-to-Work Program

• U.S. Supreme Court rules that execution of mentally retarded criminals is cruel and unusual punishment

• National Organization on Disability calls for national planning for emergencies and disaster preparedness for disability community

• College Board agrees to stop flagging scores of disabled students who take Scholastic Achievement Test (SAT) under special conditions

NOTES

INTRODUCTION

1. The Dillery case was the subject of media coverage for more than two years. See, for example, Dale Emch, "Court Reverses Conviction from Wheelchair Case," www.toledoblade.com (April 1, 2000); Kim Bates, "Ill Mother Sends Girl to Indiana," www.toledoblade.com (June 14, 1999); Kim Bates, "Wheelchair Mom Is Acquitted," www.toledoblade.com (March 12, 1999); Michael Brice, "Disability Activists Vow to Fight 'Oppression' in Sandusky," www.sanduskyregister.com (December 30, 1998). Tragically, Elias Gutierrez of Fresno, California, was killed March 18, 2001, when he was struck by a car as he was traveling next to the curb in his power wheelchair because there were no curb cuts. Gutierrez had been complaining about the lack of sidewalks with curb cuts for more than a year. Subsequently, the Fresno city council required that in all future resurfacing of streets and repair of sidewalks, curb cuts would be automatically installed if not in place. The city allocated an additional $500,000 for installing curb cuts. See "Fresno Activist Killed in Street; City Has Failed to Install Curb Cuts," *Ragged Edge* no. 4 (2001), 7; Ed Eames, "Fresno Allocates $$ for Curb Cuts in Wake of Death," *Ragged Edge* no. 1 (2002), 6.

2. H.R. 3590 (2000). The measure, known as the ADA Notification Act, was backed by the National Federation of Independent Business, the U.S. Chamber of Commerce, the National Restaurant Association, and the International Council of Shopping Centers. See "10 Years and 90 Days," *Ragged Edge* (July–August 2000), 10–13.

3. Janelle Carter, "Clint Eastwood, Disabled Spar over Disabilities Act," *Arizona Daily Sun* (May 18, 2000), 11.

4. Mary Johnson, "Eastwood Declares Loss a 'Win,'" *Ragged Edge* (November–December 2000), 25.

5. Ibid.

6. No. 99-1240.

7. Edward D. Berkowitz, *Disabled Policy: America's Programs for the Handicapped* (Cambridge: Cambridge University Press, 1987), 1.

8. Justin W. Dart, Jr., "Introduction: The ADA: A Promise to Be Kept," in *Implementing the Americans with Disabilities Act: Rights and Responsibilities of All Americans,* ed. Lawrence O. Gostin and Henry A. Beyer (Baltimore: Paul Brookes, 1993), xxi.

9. See James Anderson, *Public Policymaking*, 4th ed. (Boston: Houghton Mifflin, 2000), and John Kingdon, *Agendas, Alternatives, and Public Policies*, 2d ed. (New York: HarperCollins, 1995).

10. See Mitchell P. LaPlante, "The Demographics of Disability," *Milbank Quarterly* 69, no. 2 (winter 1991): 55–77.

11. Harlan Hahn, "Towards a Politics of Disability," *Social Science Journal* 22 (1985): 89.

12. Len Barton, "The Struggle for Citizenship: The Case of Disabled People," *Disability, Handicap and Society* 8, no. 3 (1993): 235–48.

13. On the subject of "cures" for disability, see Elliot S. Valenstein, *Great and Desperate Cures: The Rise and Decline of Psychosurgery and Other Radical Treatments for Mental Illness* (New York: Basic Books, 1986); "FDR Cured!" *Mouth* (July–August 1995), 39; Steven E. Brown, "Super Duper: The (Unfortunate) Ascendency of Christopher Reeve and the Cure-All for the 1990s," *Mainstream* 21, no. 2 (October 1996): 28–31.

14. David Pfeiffer, "Understanding Disability Policy," *Policy Studies Journal* 24, no. 1 (1996): 157–59.

15. See Paul Longmore, "A Note on Language and the Social Identity of Disabled People," *American Behavioral Scientist* 28, no. 3 (January–February 1985): 419–23.

16. Over the past ten years, an entire literature has developed around the concept of disability identity and perspectives on the oppression of disabled persons. See, for example, Max Cleland, *Strong at the Broken Places* (New York: Berkeley Books, 1980); Leah Hager Cohen, *Train Go Sorry: Inside a Deaf World* (Boston: Houghton Mifflin, 1994); Connie Panzarino, *The Me in the Mirror* (Seattle: Seal Press, 1994); Temple Grandin, *Thinking in Pictures and Other Reports from My Life with Autism* (New York: Doubleday, 1995); John Hockenberry, *Moving Violations: A Memoir* (New York: Hyperion, 1995); Elaine E. Castles, *We're People First* (Westport, Conn.: Praeger, 1996); Rosemarie Garland Thomson, *Extraordinary Bodies* (New York: Columbia University Press, 1999). For a more lighthearted view, see the work of cartoonist John Callahan (who uses a wheelchair), *Don't Worry, He Won't Get Far on Foot: The Autobiography of a Dangerous Man* (New York: William Morrow, 1989); idem, *Do Not Disturb Any Further* (New York: William Morrow, 1990); and idem, *Do What He Says! He's Crazy!!!* (New York: Quill, 1992).

17. Jane West, "The Evolution of Disability Rights," in Gostin and Beyer, *Implementing the Americans with Disabilities Act*, 10.

18. The scholarly research on disabilities is highly interdisciplinary, and this book does not attempt to begin to chronicle all the fields now considered part of "disability studies." For someone just beginning to review the literature, good sources include the various journals of the national and international associations, including *Disability Studies Quarterly* (Society for Disability Studies, published online beginning in 2002), and specialized publications such as the *Journal of Disability Policy Studies* and the international *Disability and Society*. See also Peter Monaghan, "Pioneering Field of Disability Studies Challenges Established Approaches and Attitudes," *Chronicle of Higher Education* (January 23, 1998); Elaine Makas and Lynn Schlesinger, eds., *End Results and Starting Points: Expanding the Field of Disability Studies* (Portland, Me.: Society for Disability Studies and Edmund S. Muskie Institute of Public Affairs, 1996); M. Joselyn Armstrong and Maureen H. Fitzgerald, "Culture and Disability Studies: An Anthropological Perspective," *Rehabilitation Education* 10, no. 4 (1996): 247–304; Harlan Hahn, "The Potential Impact of Disability Studies on Political Science (and Vice Versa)," *Policy Studies Journal* 21, no. 4 (1993): 740–51; and Sara D. Watson, "Introduction: Disability Policy as an Emerging Field of Mainstream Public Policy Research and Pedagogy," *Policy Studies Journal* 21, no. 4 (1993): 720–23.

Chapter 1

1. Harlan Hahn, "Civil Rights for Disabled Americans: The Foundation of a Political Agenda," in *Images of the Disabled, Disabling Images,* ed. Alan Gartner and Tom Joe (New York: Praeger, 1987), 181.

2. Ruth O'Brien, *Crippled Justice: The History of Modern Disability Policy in the Workplace* (Chicago: University of Chicago Press, 2001), 27–28.

3. National Council on the Handicapped, *National Policy for Persons with Disabilities* (Washington, D.C.: U.S. Department of Education, 1983).

4. Ibid., 181–82.

5. Ibid., 184.

6. Edward D. Berkowitz, *Disabled Policy: America's Programs for the Handicapped* (Cambridge: Cambridge University Press, 1987), 193–94.

7. William G. Johnson and Marjorie Baldwin, "The Americans with Disabilities Act: Will It Make a Difference?" *Policy Studies Journal* 21 (1993): 779.

8. See John Gliedman and William Roth, *The Unexpected Minority* (New York: Harcourt Brace Jovanovich, 1980).

9. See, for example, Edward D. Berkowitz and Monroe Berkowitz, "Widening the Field: Economics and History in the Study of Disability," *American Behavioral Scientist* 28 (January/February 1985): 405–18; Frank Bowe, *Rehabilitating America: Toward Independence for Disabled and Elderly People* (New York: Harper and Row, 1980).

10. James E. Anderson, *Public Policymaking: An Introduction,* 4th ed. (New York: Houghton Mifflin, 2000); John Kingdon, *Agendas, Alternatives, and Public Policy,* 2d ed. (Durham, N.C.: Duke University Press, 1985).

11. The work of Anderson and Kingdon is used here with the caveat that there are numerous other policy researchers and analysts whose work is similar and equally useful. In many cases, the differences in approach have more to do with the names attached to the various stages of the policy cycle than to substantive criticisms of what happens in each phase.

12. Anthony Downs, "Up and Down with Ecology—The 'Issue-Attention Cycle,'" *The Public Interest* 28 (summer 1972): 38–50.

13. See Joseph G. Morone and Edward J. Woodhouse, *Averting Catastrophe: Strategies for Regulating Risky Technologies* (Berkeley: University of California Press, 1986).

14. See Charles E. Lindblom, "The Science of 'Muddling Through,'" *Public Administration Review* 9 (1959): 79–88. See also Charles E. Lindblom and Edward J. Woodhouse, *The Policy-Making Process,* 3d ed. (New York: Prentice-Hall, 1993).

15. This issue is a prominent feature of environmental policymaking. See, for example, Jane Lubchenco, "Entering the Century of the Environment: A New Social Contract for Science," *Science* 279 (January 23, 1998): 491–97.

16. See John S. Dryzek, *Rational Ecology: Environment and Political Economy* (New York: Basil Blackwell, 1990), and idem, *Discursive Democracy: Politics, Policy, and Political Science* (Cambridge: Cambridge University Press, 1990).

17. There is an extensive literature on the topic of implementation and the factors that influence this phase of the policy process. See, for example, Robert T. Nakamura and Frank Smallwood, *The Politics of Policy Implementation* (New York: St. Martin's Press, 1980); Jeffrey Pressman and Aaron Wildavsky, *Implementation* (Berkeley: University of California Press, 1993); Daniel A. Mazmanian and Paul A. Sabatier, *Implementation and Public Policy* (Glenview, Ill.: Scott, Foresman, 1983); and Malcolm L. Goggin and others, *Implementation Theory and Practice: Toward a Third Generation* (New York: HarperCollins, 1990). On the importance of discretion in the implementation process, see, for example, Gary C. Bryner, *Bureaucratic Discretion: Law and Policy in Federal Regulatory Agencies* (New York: Pergamon Press, 1987).

18. See, for example, Robert Bartlett (ed.), *Policy through Impact Assessment: Institutionalized Analysis as a Policy Strategy* (Westport, Conn.: Greenwood Press, 1989); Eugene Meehan, *Assessing Governmental Performance* (Westport, Conn.: Greenwood Press, 1993); and Joseph Wholey and others (eds.), *Handbook of Practical Program Evaluation* (San Francisco: Jossey-Bass, 1994). These techniques have been applied to disability policy evaluation in, for example, Doria Pilling and Graham Watson (eds.), *Evaluating Quality in Services for Disabled and Older People* (Bristol, Pa.: Jessica Kingsley Publishers, 1995).

19. See, for example, Mark R. Daniels, *Terminating Public Programs: An American Political Paradox* (Armonk, N.Y.: M. E. Sharpe, 1997).

20. See Aaron Wildavsky, *Speaking Truth to Power* (Boston: Little Brown, 1979), 69–71.

21. Anderson, *Public Policymaking*, 22–23.

22. The CRD has a total of ten sections that enforce a wide range of civil and criminal statutes, including an Appellate Section and Educational Opportunities Section.

23. For a more detailed structural description of the CRD, see U.S. Commission on Civil Rights, *Helping State and Local Governments Comply with the ADA* (Washington, D.C.: U.S. Commission on Civil Rights, 1998), 6–16. The document also has a description of the section's strategic planning, implementation, and training efforts.

24. The 1964 Civil Rights Act is Public Law 88-352.

25. "HUD Creates Disability Policy Office," *Mouth* (January 1997), 5.

26. National Council on the Handicapped, *On the Threshold of Independence: A Report to the President and to the Congress* (Washington, D.C.: National Council on the Handicapped, 1988).

27. "Secretary Herman Proposes New Disability Office," press release, U.S. Department of Labor, February 9, 2000. Information on the operations of the new agency is available at www.dol.gov/odep.

28. The task force was created by Executive Order No. 13,078, 63 Fed. Reg. 13, 111 (1998).

29. "President Clinton and Vice President Gore Unveil New Initiative to Improve Economic Opportunities for Americans with Disabilities," White House press release, January 13, 1999.

30. *A Proposed Program for National Action to Combat Mental Retardation* (Washington, D.C.: President's Panel on Mental Retardation, 1962). See also Edward D. Berkowitz, "The Politics of Mental Retardation during the Kennedy Administration," *Social Science Quarterly* 61 (1980): 128–43.

31. See Richard C. Scheerenberger, *A History of Mental Retardation: A Quarter Century of Progress* (Baltimore: Paul H. Brookes, 1987), and David Braddock, *Federal Policy toward Mental Retardation and Developmental Disabilities* (Baltimore: Paul H. Brookes, 1987).

32. Public Law 98-221.

33. The National Council on Disability has a website that can be accessed at www.ncd.gov.

34. National Council on the Handicapped, *Toward Independence: An Assessment of Federal Laws and Programs Affecting People with Disabilities, with Legislative Recommendations* (Washington, D.C.: National Council on the Handicapped, 1986).

35. *From ADA to Empowerment: The Report of the Task Force on the Rights and Empowerment of Americans with Disabilities* (Washington, D.C.: Task Force on the Rights and Empowerment of Americans with Disabilities, 1990).

36. Ibid., 24. In late 1998, for instance, the DRS had only fifteen investigators to respond to complaints from the entire United States.

37. Ibid., 24–25.

38. C.F.R., Section 35.176 .1997.

39. See, for example, Ed and Toni Eames, "The Department of Justice and Us," *Ragged Edge* (September–October 1998), 12–14, 17.

CHAPTER 2

1. Jane Richardson Hanks and Lucien M. Hanks, Jr., "The Physically Handicapped in Certain Non-Occidental Societies," *Journal of Social Issues* 13 (1948): 11–20.

2. Simi Linton, *Claiming Disability: Knowledge and Identity* (New York: New York University Press, 1998), 22–23.

3. Robert Funk, "Disability Rights: From Caste to Class in the Context of Civil Rights," in *Images of the Disabled, Disabling Images,* ed. Alan Gartner and Tom Joe (New York: Praeger, 1987), 9–23.

4. For additional historical commentary on the freak show phenomenon, see Robert Bogdan, *Freak Show: Presenting Human Oddities for Amusement and Profit* (Chicago: University of Chicago Press, 1988); Frederick Drimmer, *Very Special People: The Struggles, Loves and Triumphs of Human Oddities* (New York: Bantam Books, 1973); Leslie Fiedler, *Freaks: Myths and Images of the Secret Self* (New York: Simon and Schuster, 1978).

5. Claire H. Liachowitz, *Disability as a Social Construct: Legislative Roots* (Philadelphia: University of Pennsylvania Press, 1988), 67–68.

6. See Harlan Lane, *When the Mind Hears: A History of the Deaf* (New York: Random House, 1984).

7. See C. W. Bledsoe, "Dr. Samuel Gridley Howe and the Family Tree of Residential Schools," *Journal of Visual Impairment and Blindness* 87 (1993): 174–76; Milton Meltzer, *A Light in the Dark: The Life of Samuel Gridley Howe* (New York: Crowell, 1964); Laura E. Howe Richards, *Two Noble Lives* (Boston: D. Estes and Co., 1911); Harold Schwartz, *Samuel Gridley Howe: Social Reformer* (Cambridge, Mass.: Harvard University Press, 1956).

8. See Dorothy Clarke Wilson, *Stranger and Traveler: The Story of Dorothea Dix, American Reformer* (Boston: Little Brown, 1975).

9. Richard K. Scotch, *From Good Will to Civil Rights: Transforming Federal Disability Policy* (Philadelphia: Temple University Press, 1984), 16.

10. Clifford W. Beers, *A Mind that Found Itself* (New York: Doubleday, 1965).

11. See also Roy Porter, *A Social History of Madness: The World through the Eyes of the Insane* (New York: Dutton, 1989).

12. James W. Trent, Jr., *Inventing the Feeble Mind: A History of Mental Retardation in the United States* (Berkeley: University of California Press, 1994),

13–15. For more on Sequin, see Henry Holman, *Sequin and His Physiological Method of Education* (London: Pitman and Sons, 1914), and Linus P. Brockett, "The Sequin Physiological School," *New York Times* (October 29, 1882). Sequin's theories can be found (in English) in Edouard Sequin, *Idiocy and its Treatment by the Physiological Method* (New York: W. Wood, 1866).

13. Linus P. Brockett, "Idiots and Institutions for their Training," *American Journal of Education* I (1855): 593–608, and idem, "Cretins and Idiots: What Has Been Done and What Can Be Done for Them," *Atlantic Monthly* (January 1858), 410–19. See also Martin W. Barr, *Mental Defectives: Their History, Treatment, and Training* (Philadelphia: Blakiston Press, 1904).

14. Trent, *Inventing the Feeble Mind*, 162.

15. Henry H. Goddard, *The Kallikak Family: A Study in the Heredity of Feeble-Mindedness* (New York: Macmillan, 1912). See also J. David Smith, *Minds Made Feeble: The Myth and Legacy of the Kallikaks* (Rockville, Md.: Aspen Systems Corp., 1985). For more on Henry Goddard and his own legacy, see Leila Zenderland, *Measuring Minds: Henry Herbert Goddard and the Origins of American Intelligence Testing* (Cambridge: Cambridge University Press, 1998).

16. Richard L. Dugdale, *The Jukes: A Study in Crime, Pauperism, Disease, and Heredity* (New York: Putnam, 1877). See also Arthur H. Estabrook, *The Jukes in 1915* (Washington, D.C.: Carnegie Institution, 1916), and Alfred E. Winship, *Jukes-Edwards: A Study in Education and Heredity* (Harrisburg, Pa.: R. L. Myers, 1900).

17. Arthur H. Estabrook and Charles B. Davenport, *The Nam Family: A Study in Cacogenics* (Cold Spring Harbor, N.Y.: Press of the New Era, 1912).

18. See, for example, Charles B. Davenport and Florence Danielson, *The Hill Folk: Report on a Rural Community of Hereditary Defectives* (Cold Spring Harbor, N.Y.: Press of the New Era, 1912); Arthur H. Estabrook and Ivan E. MacDougle, *Mongrel Virginians: The Win Tribe* (Baltimore: Williams and Wilkins, 1926); Mary S. Kostir, *Family of Sam Sixty* (Mansfield: Press of the Ohio State Reformatory, 1916).

19. Trent, *Inventing the Feeble Mind*, 6.

20. Ibid., 168. See also John Higham, *Strangers in the Land: Patterns of American Nativism 1860–1925* (New York: Atheneum, 1963).

21. Sir Francis Galton, *Inquiries into Human Faculty and its Development* (London: Macmillan, 1893). See also Charles Davenport, *Heredity in Relation to Eugenics* (New York: Henry Holt, 1911), and Daniel J. Kevles, *In the Name of Eugenics: Genetics and the Use of Human Heredity* (New York: Knopf, 1985).

22. In Nazi Germany, the code name T-4 was used during the early 1940s to describe the extermination of persons Adolph Hitler called the "useless eaters." Hitler had given an order that gave physicians authority to euthanize adults with disabilities at designated psychiatric hospitals or nursing homes; others were murdered in concentration camps. Disabled children had to be registered with the government, and many were starved to death in the more than thirty

institutions charged with their care. See Hugh Gregory Gallagher, *By Trust Betrayed: Patients, Physicians, and the License to Kill in the Third Reich* (New York: Henry Holt, 1990); Robert Proctor, *Racial Hygiene: Medicine under the Nazis* (Cambridge, Mass.: Harvard University Press, 1988); Robert Jay Lifton, *The Nazi Doctors: Medical Killing and the Psychology of Genocide* (New York: Basic Books, 1986).

23. Fred Pelka, *The ABC-CLIO Companion to the Disability Rights Movement* (Santa Barbara, Calif.: ABC-CLIO, 1997), 115.

24. Beatrice Ann Posner Wright, *Physical Disability: A Psychosocial Approach*, 2d ed. (New York: Harper and Row, 1983).

25. Kenneth M. Stampp, *The Era of Reconstruction 1865–1877* (New York: Knopf, 1965).

26. See, for example, Timothy M. Cook, "The Americans with Disabilities Act: The Move to Integration," *Temple Law Review* 64 (1991): 393–469.

27. Walter Fernald, "The Burden of Feeblemindedness," *Journal of Psychoasthenics* 18 (1912): 90–98, quoted in David Pfeiffer, "Overview of the Disability Movement: History, Legislative Record, and Political Implications," *Policy Studies Journal* 21 (1993): 726.

28. For a review of the practice, see Stephen Trombley, *The Right to Reproduce: A History of Coercive Sterilization* (London: Weidenfeld and Nicolson, 1988); and Philip R. Reilly, *The Surgical Solution: A History of Involuntary Sterilization in the United States* (Baltimore: Johns Hopkins University Press, 1991).

29. Opinion of Chief Justice Oliver Wendell Holmes in *Buck v. Bell*, 274 U.S. 200 (1927). For two contrasting perspectives, see Leon Whitney, *The Case for Sterilization* (New York: Frederick A. Stokes, 1934), and J. David Smith and K. Ray Nelson, *The Sterilization of Carrie Buck* (Far Hills, N.J.: New Horizon Press, 1989).

30. E. Z. Ferster, "Eliminating the Unfit: Is Sterilization the Answer?" *Ohio State Law Journal* 27 (1966): 591–63.

31. See Susan J. Spungin, *Braille Literacy: Issues for Blind Persons, Families, Professionals, and Producers of Braille* (New York: American Foundation for the Blind, 1989).

32. See Arden Neisser, *The Other Side of Silence: Sign Language and the Deaf Community in America* (New York: Knopf, 1983), and Richard Winefield, *Never the Twain Shall Meet: Bell, Gallaudet, and the Communications Debate* (Washington, D.C.: Gallaudet University Press, 1987).

33. Mary Jane Ward, *The Snake Pit* (New York: Random House, 1946).

34. Burton Blatt and Fred Kaplan, *Christmas in Purgatory* (New York: Allyn and Bacon, 1966).

35. Nancy R. Weiss, *The Application of Aversive Procedures to Individuals with Developmental Disabilities: A Call to Action* (Seattle: Association for Persons with Severe Handicaps, 1991).

36. The best account of the events leading up to the incident can be found in David and Sheila Rothman's *The Willowbrook Wars: A Decade of Struggle for Social Change* (New York: Harper and Row, 1984). See also the writings of the man who brought Willowbrook to the public's attention: Geraldo Rivera, *Willowbrook: A Report on How It Is and Why It Doesn't Have To Be That Way* (New York: Random House, 1972).

37. See Richard C. Scheerenberger, *Deinstitutionalization and Institutional Reform* (Springfield, Ill.: Charles C. Thomas, 1976).

38. President's Panel on Mental Retardation (1962).

39. See, for example, *Pennhurst State School and Hospital v. Halderman*, 451 U.S. 1 (1981), and *O'Connor v. Donaldson*, 422 U.S. 563 (1975), in which the U.S. Supreme Court ruled that people with psychiatric disabilities who were not dangerous to themselves or others could not be incarcerated against their will.

40. Joseph Shapiro, "Disability Policy and the Media: A Stealth Civil Rights Movement Bypasses the Press and Defies Conventional Wisdom," *Policy Studies Journal* 22 (1994): 124.

41. Ibid.

42. Douglas Biklen and Robert Bogdan, "Media Portrayals of Disabled People: A Study in Stereotypes," *Interracial Books for Children Bulletin* 4, no. 6 (1982): 7. See also Beth Haller, "Rethinking Models of Media Representation of Disability," *Disability Studies Quarterly* 15, no. 2 (spring 1995): 35–48; Zenaida Sarabia Panol and Michael McBride, "Disability Images in Print Advertising: Exploring Attitudinal Impact Issues," *Disability Studies Quarterly* 21, no. 2 (spring 2001), available at www.cds.hawaii.edu/dsq (accessed May 21, 2001); Beth Haller and Sue Ralph, "Profitability, Diversity, and Disability Images in Advertising," *Disability Studies Quarterly* 21, no. 2 (spring 2001), available at www.cds.hawaii.edu/dsq (accessed May 21, 2001).

43. See, for example, "What a High-Powered Agent Can Do for You," *Ragged Edge* (July–August 2000), 25. The article describes Harvard University student Brooke Ellison, who is being represented by the prestigious William Morris talent agency in writing her autobiography.

44. Jack A. Nelson, "Broken Images: Portrayals of Those with Disabilities in American Media," in *The Disabled, the Media, and the Information Age*, ed. Jack A. Nelson (Westport, Conn.: Greenwood Press, 1994), 4–9.

45. Scotch, *From Good Will to Civil Rights*, 28.

CHAPTER 3

1. Robert Haveman and others, *Public Policy toward Disabled Workers* (Ithaca, N.Y.: Cornell University Press, 1984).

2. Ibid.

3. Edward D. Berkowitz, *Disabled Policy: America's Programs for the Handicapped* (Cambridge: Cambridge University Press, 1987), 1953.

4. Claire H. Liachowitz, *Disability as a Social Construct: Legislative Roots* (Philadelphia: University of Pennsylvania Press, 1988), 19–20.

5. For a discussion of the role of the disabled soldier in the Civil War, see Bruce Catton, *A Stillness at Appomattox* (New York: Doubleday, 1953).

6. Gary L. Albrecht, *The Disability Business: Rehabilitation in America* (Newbury Park, Calif.: Sage Publications, 1992), 98.

7. Berkowitz, *Disabled Policy*, 15.

8. For a historical perspective, see, for example, Walter Dodd, *Administration of Workmen's Compensation* (New York: Commonwealth Fund, 1936); Herman M. Somers and Anne Somers, *Workmen's Compensation: Prevention, Insurance and Rehabilitation of Occupational Disability* (New York: John Wiley, 1954); David Appal and John D. Warhol, eds., *Workers' Compensation Benefits: Adequacy, Equity, and Efficiency* (Ithaca, N.Y.: ICR Press, 1985).

9. There is considerable commentary about the development of American social security programs from the initial development of federal statutes through the 1980s. See, for example, Edwin E. Witte, *The Development of the Social Security Act* (Madison: University of Wisconsin Press, 1962); Robert M. Ball, *Social Security: Today and Tomorrow* (New York: Columbia University Press, 1978); Martha Derthick, *Policymaking for Social Security* (Washington, D.C.: Brookings Institution Press, 1979); Deborah Stone, *The Disabled State* (Philadelphia: Temple University Press, 1984); Robert J. Myers, *Social Security* (Homewood, Ill.: Richard D. Irwin, 1985); W. Andrew Achenbaum, *Social Security: Visions and Revisions* (Cambridge: Cambridge University Press, 1986).

10. This definition is quoted in Arthur Altmeyer, "Social Insurance for Permanently Disabled Workers," *Social Security Bulletin* (March 1941): 4. See also Arthur J. Altmeyer, *The Formative Years of Social Security* (Madison: University of Wisconsin Press, 1966).

11. Berkowitz, *Disabled Policy*, 46.

12. Ibid., 66.

13. Richard V. Burkhauser, Robert H. Haveman, and Barbara L. Wolfe, "How People with Disabilities Fare When Public Policies Change," *Journal of Policy Analysis and Management* 12, no. 2 (1993): 251–69.

14. See *More Diligent Followup Needed to Weed Out Ineligible SSA Disability Beneficiaries* (Washington, D.C.: U.S. General Accounting Office, 1982).

15. Berkowitz, *Disabled Policy*, 126–27.

16. Ibid., 256. See also Caroline L. Weaver, "Social Security Disability Policy in the 1980s and Beyond," in *Disability and the Labor Market: Economic Problems, Policy and Programs,* ed. Monroe Berkowitz and M. A. Hill (Ithaca, N.Y.: RLR Press, 1986), 29–63.

17. For an analysis of the social security reform movement, see Susan G. Mezey, *No Longer Disabled: The Federal Courts and the Politics of Social Security Disability* (Westport, Conn.: Greenwood Press, 1988).

18. Berkowitz, *Disabled Policy*, 151.

19. See Douglas C. McMurtie, *The Disabled Soldier* (New York: Macmillan, 1919).

20. Liachowitz, *Disability as a Social Construct*, 38.

21. Berkowitz, *Disabled Policy*, 153.

22. Beatrice A. Wright, *Physical Disability: A Psychological Approach* (New York: Harper and Row, 1960), 38.

23. Public Law 93-112; 29 U.S.C. Section 700 *et seq.*

24. Liachowitz, *Disability as a Social Construct*, 40.

25. Ibid., 82. For a comprehensive overview, see C. Esco Obermann, *A History of Vocational Rehabilitation in America* (Minneapolis: Denison, 1965); Blanche D. Coll, *Perspectives in Public Welfare* (Washington, D.C.: Department of Health, Education, and Welfare, 1969); James Bitter, *Introduction to Rehabilitation* (St. Louis: C. V. Mosby, 1979).

26. Berkowitz, *Disabled Policy*, 176.

27. *Vocational Rehabilitation: Your Key to an Independent Future* (Washington, D.C.: Department of Veterans Affairs, Veterans Benefits Administration, 1990).

28. The three audits are *VA Can Provide More Employment Assistance to Vets Who Complete Its Vocational Rehabilitation Program, Better VA Management Needed to Help Disabled Veterans Find Jobs*; and *Vocational Rehabilitation: VA Continues to Place Few Disabled Veterans* (Washington, D.C.: U.S. Government Accounting Office, 1984, 1992, 1996).

29. Gary F. Holmes, "The Historical Roots of the Empowerment Dilemma in Vocational Rehabilitation," *Journal of Disability Policy Studies* 4, no. 1 (1993): 2–63.

30. Statement of Senator Hubert Humphrey to U.S. Senate, *Congressional Record,* 20 January 1972, 526.

31. Richard K. Scotch, *From Good Will to Civil Rights: Transforming Federal Disability Policy* (Philadelphia: Temple University Press, 1984), 44.

32. See Frank G. Bowe, *Handicapping America: Barriers to Disabled People* (New York: Harper and Row, 1978). The legislation became Public Law 93-112.

33. Stephen L. Percy, "ADA, Disability Rights, and Evolving Regulatory Federalism," *Publius* 23 (fall 1993): 90.

34. National Council on the Handicapped, *Toward Independence: An Assessment of Federal Laws and Programs Affecting Persons with Disabilities* (Washington, D.C.: National Council on the Handicapped, 1986), 7.

35. Scotch, *From Good Will to Civil Rights*, 53.

36. U.S. 397 (1979). See also Betsy Shrauder and Jeannine Villing, eds., *Proceedings of the Supreme Court Davis Decision: Implications for Higher Education and Physically Disabled Students* (Detroit, Mich.: Wayne State University, 1979).

37. See Douglas Biklen, *Let Our Children Go: An Organizing Manual for Advocates and Parents* (Syracuse, N.Y.: Human Policy Press, 1974).

38. Public Law 94-142, U.S.C. Section 1232.

39. See Janet Duncan and Kathy Hulgin, *Resources on Inclusive Education* (Syracuse, N.Y.: Research Training Center, 1993), and Jacqueline Thousand and Richard A. Villa, *Creating an Inclusive School* (Alexandria, Va.: Association for Supervision and Curriculum Development, 1995).

40. U.S.C. Section 1400 *et seq.*

41. David Tilbury, "Advocates at Rally Vent Frustration with Special Education," *Ragged Edge* (January–February 1999), 8.

42. Dave Reynbolds, "Schools to Be Penalized on Education Ruling," *Ragged Edge* no. 3 (2001), 14.

43. Albrecht, *The Disability Business*, 134–37.

44. Ibid., 141.

45. There are more economic and management perspectives on the disability business than policy case studies. See, for example, Mark Priestly, *Disability Politics and Community Care* (London: Jessica Kingsley Publishers, 1999), and Raymond C. O'Brien and Michael T. Flannery, *Long-Term Care: Federal, State, and Private Options for the Future* (New York: Haworth Press, 1997). For a case study approach, see Julie Ann Racino, "Organizational Case Studies: Creating Change in Housing, Employment, Families, and Community Support," in *Policy, Program Evaluation, and Research in Disability,* ed. Julie Ann Racino (New York: Haworth Press, 1999), 315–34.

46. Albrecht, *The Disability Business*, 141.

CHAPTER 4

1. Lillie S. Ransom, "How Deaf Students Won Their Case at Gallaudet University—by Taking to the Streets," in *The Disabled, the Media, and the Information Age,* ed. Jack A. Nelson (Westport, Conn.: Greenwood Press, 1994), 147–57.

2. John B. Christiansen and Sharon N. Barnartt, *Deaf President Now! The 1988 Revolution at Gallaudet University* (Washington, D.C.: Gallaudet University Press, 1995), 215. See also Jack Gannon, *The Week the World Heard Gallaudet* (Washington, D.C.: Gallaudet University Press, 1989); Sean Picolli, "Alumni, Faculty Group Presses Gallaudet to Pick Deaf President," *Washington Times* (December 28, 1987), 1.

3. David S. Meyer and Sidney G. Tarrow, *The Social Movement Society* (Oxford: Rowman and Littlefield, 1998).

4. See, for example, J. Freeman, *Social Movements of the Sixties and Seventies* (New York: Longman, 1983), and John D. McCarthy and Mayer N. Zald, *The Trend of Social Movements in America: Professionalism and Resource Mobilization* (Morristown, N.J.: General Learning Press, 1973).

5. Ralph H. Turner and Lewis M. Killian, *Collective Behavior* (New York: Prentice-Hall, 1987). See also Neil S. Smelser, *Theory of Collective Behavior* (New York: Free Press, 1962).

6. This contrarian view is offered by Walter K. Olson, *The Excuse Factory: How Employment Law Is Paralyzing the American Workplace* (New York: Free Press, 1997), 94–95.

7. Richard K. Scotch, "Politics and Policy in the History of the Disability Rights Movement," *Milbank Quarterly* 67, suppl. 2, pt. 2 (1989): 380–400.

8. Ibid., 382–83.

9. Earl Latham, *The Group Basis of Politics* (New York: Octagon Books, 1965).

10. David Easton, *A Systems Analysis of Political Life* (New York: Wiley, 1965).

11. The classic literature on rational choice and similar theories includes Mancur Olson, *The Logic of Collective Action* (Cambridge, Mass.: Harvard University Press, 1965); David Truman, *The Governmental Process* (New York: Knopf, 1962); James Q. Wilson, *Political Organizations* (New York: Basic Books, 1973); Anthony Downs, *An Economic Theory of Democracy* (New York: Harper and Row, 1957).

12. Scotch, "Politics and Policy," 384.

13. See, for example, Paul Longmore, "Uncovering the Hidden History of People with Disabilities," *Reviews in American History* 15 (September 1987): 355–64; Irving Howards, Henry P. Brehm, and Saad Z. Nagi, *Disability: From Social Problem to Federal Program* (New York: Praeger, 1980); Paul Longmore, "The Second Phase: From Disability Rights to Disability Culture," *Disability Rag and Resource* 16, no. 5 (September–October 1995): 4–11.

14. See, for example, Barrett Shaw, ed., *The Ragged Edge: The Disability Experience from the Pages of the First Fifteen Years of* The Disability Rag (Louisville, Ky.: Advocado Press, 1994); Nora Ellen Groce, *The U.S. Role in International Disability Activities: A History and a Look toward the Future* (Oakland, Calif.: World Institute on Disability, 1992); Marilyn Golden, "Damn Straight We're a Real Movement!" *Disability Rag and Resource* 17, no. 2 (March–April 1996): 1, 4–5, 15; John Hockenberry, *Moving Violations, a Memoir: War Zones, Wheelchairs, and Declarations of Independence* (New York: Hyperion, 1995); Cyndi Jones, "20 Years: We've Come a Long Way," *Mainstream* 20, no. 6 (March 1996): 17–21.

15. See, for example, Steve Taylor and Stan Searl, "The Disabled in America: History, Policy and Trends," in *Understanding Exceptional Children and Youth,* ed. Peter Knoblock (Boston: Little Brown, 1987), 5–64.

16. James I. Charlton, *Nothing about Us without Us: Disability Oppression and Empowerment* (Berkeley: University of California Press, 1998), 136–48.

17. Carl Boggs, *Social Movements and Political Power* (Philadelphia: Temple University Press, 1986).

18. See Gerben DeJong, *Environmental Accessibility and Independent Living Outcomes* (East Lansing, Mich.: University Center for International Rehabilitation, 1981); Barry Bernstein, *Challenges of Emerging Leadership:*

Community-Based Independent Living Programs and the Disability Rights Movement (Washington, D.C.: Institute for Educational Leadership, 1984).

19. There is a substantial literature on the independent living movement, which now encompasses more than 400 advocacy centers in the United States. See, for example, Nancy M. Crewe and Irving Kenneth Zola, eds., *Independent Living for Physically Disabled People* (San Francisco: Jossey-Bass, 1983); Chava W. Levy, *A People's History of the Independent Living Movement* (Lawrence, Kans.: Research and Training Center on Independent Living, 1988); Diane Driedge, *The Last Civil Rights Movement: Disabled Peoples' International* (New York: St. Martin's Press, 1989), 28; Fred Pelka, "Ed Roberts, 1939–1995," *Mainstream* (May 1995); Julie Ann Racino, *Living in the Community: Toward Supportive Policies in Housing and Community Services* (Syracuse, N.Y.: Community and Policy Studies, 1993), 20; Devva Kasnitz, "Life Event Histories and the U.S. Independent Living Movement," in *Disability and the Life Course,* ed. M. Priestly (Cambridge: Cambridge University Press, 2001), 67–79.

20. Kasnitz, "Life Event Histories."

21. Charlton, *Nothing about Us without Us*, 17.

22. Joseph P. Shapiro, *No Pity: People with Disabilities Forging a New Civil Rights Movement* (New York: Random House, 1993), 126.

23. See Keith Fitzgerald, "The Politics of Plagues: Responses to the AIDS Epidemic in Historical Perspective," *Journal of Policy History* 8, no. 2 (1996): 253–59.

24. Ibid., 237.

25. See James R. Tompkins, *Child Advocacy: History, Theory, and Practice* (Durham, N.C.: Academic Press, 1998); Joseph M. Hawes, *The Children's Rights Movement: A History of Advocacy and Protection* (Boston: Twayne Publishers, 1991); H. Rutherford Turnbull and Ann P. Turnbull, *Parents Speak Out: Then and Now* (Columbus, Ohio: Charles E. Merrill, 1985); Philip L. Safford, *A History of Childhood and Disability* (New York: Teachers College Press, 1996).

26. Charlton, *Nothing about Us without Us,* 121.

27. See, for example, the analysis of Frances Fox Piven and Richard A. Cloward, *Poor People's Movements: Why They Succeed, How They Fail* (New York: Random House, 1979); Michael Lipsky, "Protest as a Political Resource," *American Political Science Review* 62 (1968): 1144–58; Jerry Rose, *Outbreaks: The Sociology of Collective Behavior* (New York: Free Press, 1982).

28. Scotch, *Politics and Policy,* 388.

29. ADAPT has changed the meaning of its acronym; it is now American Disabled for Attendant Programs Today—emphasizing its new focus on personal attendant services.

30. Mary Johnson and Barrett Shaw, eds., *To Ride the Public's Buses: The Fight that Built a Movement* (Louisville, Ky.: Advocado Press, 2001).

31. Ibid., 4–6.

32. For more on the historical background of ADAPT, see Laura Hershey, "Wade Blank's Liberated Community," in *The Ragged Edge: The Disability Experience from the Pages of the First Fifteen Years of* The Disability Rag, ed. Barrett Shaw (Louisville, Ky.: Advocado Press, 1994).

33. Shapiro, *No Pity*, 135.

34. "Disabled Shut Down Health and Human Services," ADAPT press release, November 3, 1998 (adaptpr@dnet.acils.com).

35. Manny Fernandez, "Protest over Access on Greyhound Buses: Ramps Needed, Wheelchair Users Say," *San Francisco Chronicle* (January 16, 1998), A16.

36. Charles Tilly, "Speaking Your Mind without Elections, Surveys or Social Movements," *Public Opinion Quarterly* 47 (1983): 461–78.

37. Douglas P. Biklen, *Community Organizing: Theory and Practice* (New York: Prentice-Hall, 1983).

38. Christiansen and Barnartt, *Deaf President Now!* 173.

39. Shapiro, *No Pity*, 128.

40. Scotch, *Politics and Policy*, 389.

41. Ibid., 177.

42. David L. Miller, *Introduction to Collective Behavior* (Prospect Heights, Ill.: Waveland Press, 1985).

43. See Richard Scotch, *From Good Will to Civil Rights: Transforming Federal Disability Policy* (Philadelphia: Temple University Press, 1984).

44. Martin Weil, "Gallaudet Student Awarded $1,500 in McDonald's Case," *Washington Post* (December 31, 1997), B2.

45. Public Law 94-103.

46. U.S.C. Section 732.

47. U.S.C. Section 794e.

48. Jane West, Introduction, in Jane West, ed., *Implementing the Americans with Disabilities Act* (Cambridge, Mass.: Blackwell Publishers, 1996), 20–21.

49. Paul K. Longmore and David Goldberger, "The League of the Physically Handicapped and the Great Depression: A Case Study in New Disability History," *Journal of American History* 87, no. 3 (December 2000); available at www.historycoop.org/journals/jah (accessed February 28, 2001).

50. Ibid.

51. Ibid.

CHAPTER 5

1. Justin W. Dart, Jr., "Introduction: The ADA: A Promise to Be Kept," in *Implementing the Americans with Disabilities Act: Rights and Responsibilities of All Americans,* ed. Lawrence O. Gostin and Henry A. Beyer (Baltimore: Paul H. Brookes, 1993), xxii.

2. Justin W. Dart, Jr., speaking to Easter Seals Project ACTION Roundtable on Measuring the Benefits of Accessible Transportation, Alexandria, Virginia, September 19, 2000.

3. "Justin Dart: 1930–2002," www.thearclink.org/news/article (June 23, 2002).

4. Joseph P. Shapiro, *No Pity: People with Disabilities Forging a New Civil Rights Movement* (New York: Random House, 1993), 141–42.

5. National Council on the Handicapped, *Toward Independence: An Assessment of Federal Laws and Programs Affecting Persons with Disabilities, with Legislative Recommendations* (Washington, D.C.: National Council on the Handicapped, 1986).

6. National Council on Disability, *On the Threshold of Independence* (Washington, D.C.: National Council on Disability, 1988).

7. Susan F. Rasky, "How the Disabled Sold Congress on a New Bill of Rights," *New York Times* (September 17, 1989), 5.

8. John W. Kingdon, *Agendas, Alternatives, and Public Policies,* 2d ed. (New York: HarperCollins, 1995), 165.

9. Ibid.

10. Ibid., 167.

11. Sara D. Watson, "A Study in Legislative Strategy: The Passage of the ADA," in Gostin and Beyer, *Implementing the Americans with Disabilities Act,* 26.

12. Arlene Mayerson, "The History of the ADA: A Movement Perspective," in Gostin and Beyer, *Implementing the Americans with Disabilities Act,* 17–24. Another activist's view can be found in Jan Little, *If It Weren't for the Honor, I Would Have Walked: Previously Untold Tales of the Journey to the ADA* (Cambridge, Mass.: Brookline Books, 1996).

13. See Leonard W. Weiss and Michael W. Klass, eds., *Regulatory Reform: What Really Happened* (Boston: Little, Brown, 1986).

14. See C. R. Babcock, "Handicapped Policy Undergoing a Rewrite," *Washington Post* (March 4, 1982), A27.

15. Although the term is somewhat generic, it is used by researcher Jane West in her article "The Evolution of Disability Rights," in Gostin and Beyer, *Implementing the Americans with Disabilities Act,* 10.

16. U.S.C. Sections 4151–4157 (1968).

17. U.S.C. Section 6000–6081 (1975).

18. U.S.C. Section 1997 *et seq.* (1980).

19. P.L. 100-259, 20 U.S.C. Section 168 *et seq.*, 29 U.S.C. Section 706, 42 U.S.C. Section 2000 (1988).

20. Mayerson, "The History of the ADA," 22.

21. Watson, "A Study in Legislative Strategy," 28.

22. Letters included in *Congressional Record—Senate* by Senator Edward Kennedy, September 7, 1989.

23. For a discussion of this issue, see, for example, L. D. Brown, "Civil Rights and Regulatory Wrongs: The Reagan Administration and the Medical Treatment of Handicapped Infants," *Journal of Health Policy, Politics and Law* 11, no. 2 (1986): 231–54.

24. Richard K. Scotch, "Politics and Policy in the History of the Disability Rights Movement." *Milbank Quarterly* 67, suppl. 2, pt. 2 (1989): 396–97.

25. Testimony of Senator David Pryor, *Congressional Record—Senate*, September 7, 1989, 19840.

26. Shapiro, *No Pity*, 119-125.

27. Testimony of Senator Orrin Hatch, *Congressional Record—Senate*, September 7, 1989, 19836.

28. Testimony of Senator Tom Harkin, *Congressional Record—Senate*, September 7, 1989, 19847.

29. James Bovard, "The Lame Game," *American Spectator* (July 1995), 30–33.

30. "The Lawyers' Employment Act," *Wall Street Journal* (September 11, 1989), A18.

31. Testimony of Senator Edward Kennedy, *Congressional Record—Senate*, September 7, 1989, 19888.

32. Martin Linsky, "The Media and Public Deliberation," in *The Power of Public Ideas,* ed. R. B. Reich (Cambridge, Mass.: Ballinger, 1988), 205–27.

33. Joseph P. Shapiro, "Disability Rights as Civil Rights: The Struggle for Recognition," in *The Disabled, the Media, and the Information Age,* ed. Jack A. Nelson (Westport, Conn.: Greenwood Press, 1994), 59.

34. Ibid.

35. Joseph P. Shapiro, "Disability Policy and the Media: A Stealth Civil Rights Movement Bypasses the Press and Defies Conventional Wisdom," *Policy Studies Journal* 22, no. 1 (1994): 131.

36. Watson, "A Study in Legislative Strategy," 28.

37. See Fred Pelka, "Bashing the Disabled: The Right Wing Attack on the ADA," *The Humanist* (November–December 1996), 26–30.

38. Letter from John J. Motley III, National Federation of Independent Business, to Senator Orrin Hatch, *Congressional Record—Senate*, September 7, 1989, 19841.

39. Testimony from the representatives of these organizations appears in "Americans with Disabilities Act of 1989," hearings before Subcommittee on Civil and Constitutional Rights, House Judiciary Committee, October 11, 1989, 80–151.

40. Two days of subcommittee hearings were held on these issues, serialized in "Americans with Disabilities Act," hearings before Subcommittee on Surface Transportation, House Public Works and Transportation Committee, September 20, 26, 1989.

41. Address of President George Bush at signing of Americans with Disabilities Act, July 26, 1990.

Chapter 6

1. Justin W. Dart, Jr., "The ADA: A Promise To Be Kept," in *Implementing the Americans with Disabilities Act: Rights and Responsibilities of All Americans,* ed. Lawrence O. Gostin and Henry A. Beyer (Baltimore: Paul H. Brookes, 1993), xxiv.

2. See, for example, Peter C. Bishop and Augustus J. Jones, Jr., "Implementing the Americans with Disabilities Act of 1990: Assessing the Variables of Success," *Public Administration Review* 53, no. 2 (March–April 1993): 121–28; Frederick C. Collignon, "Is the ADA Successful? Indicators for Tracking Gains," *Annals of the American Academy of Political and Social Sciences* 549 (January 1997): 129–47; Leslie Pickering Francis and Anita Silvers, eds., *Americans with Disabilities: Exploring Implications of the Law for Individuals and Institutions* (New York: Routledge, 2000); Jacqueline Vaughn Switzer, ed., "Symposium: The ADA: Ten Years Later," *Policy Studies Journal* 29, no. 4 (2001). This symposium is a series of articles that deal with perspectives on various provisions of the ADA, commissioned for the tenth anniversary of the statute's signing.

3. A person with a disability has 300 days to file a complaint if it is done with a designated state or local fair employment practice agency.

4. There is a substantial, and often conflicting, body of early literature on implementation as a step in the policymaking process. See, for example, Charles O. Jones, *An Introduction to the Study of Public Policy* (Belmont, Calif.: Wadsworth, 1970); Jeffrey Pressman and Aaron Wildavsky, *Implementation* (Berkeley: University of California Press, 1973); T. B. Smith, "The Policy Implementation Process," *Policy Sciences* 4 (1973): 197–209; Donald Van Meter and Carl Van Horn, "The Policy Implementation Process: A Conceptual Framework," *Administration and Society* 6, no. 4 (February 1975): 445–88; Eugene Bardach, *The Implementation Game: What Happens after a Bill Becomes a Law* (Cambridge, Mass.: MIT Press, 1977); Robert T. Nakamura and Frank Smallwood, *The Politics of Policy Implementation* (New York: St. Martin's Press, 1980); George C. Edwards, *Implementing Public Policy* (Washington, D.C.: Congressional Quarterly Press, 1980). In addition, there are numerous case studies to which these conceptual models apply.

5. Jane West, "The Federal Government and Congress," in *Implementing the Americans with Disabilities Act,* ed. Jane West (Cambridge, Mass.: Blackwell Publishers, 1996), 5.

6. Andrew I. Batavia, "Ten Years Later: The ADA and the Future of Disability Policy," in Francis and Silvers, *Americans with Disabilities*, 283.

7. *Federal Register*, July 26, 1991, 35727.

8. *Federal Register*, July 26, 1991.

9. Ibid., 35694–35695.

10. American National Standards Institute, *American Standard Specifications for Making Buildings and Facilities Accessible to, and Usable by, the Physically Handicapped* (New York: American National Standards Institute, 1961).

11. U.S. General Accounting Office, *Further Action Needed to Make All Buildings Accessible to the Physically Handicapped* (Washington, D.C.: U.S. General Accounting Office, 1975).

12. Stephen L. Percy, *Disability, Civil Rights, and Public Policy: The Politics of Implementation* (Tuscaloosa: University of Alabama Press, 1989).

13. U.S. General Accounting Office, *Further Action Needed*, 6, 27–28.

14. Regulatory negotiation became a popular tool during the Clinton administration. See, for example, Patrick Fn'Piere and Linda Work, "On the Growth and Development of Dispute Resolution," *Kentucky Law Journal* 81 (1992–1993): 959–75; Cindy Skrzycki, "Finding Common Ground in the Middle of the Table, *Washington Post* (February 23, 1996), B1; Edward P. Weber and Anne M. Khademian, "From Agitation to Collaboration: Clearing the Air through Negotiation," *Public Administration Review* 57, no. 5 (September–October 1997): 396–410.

15. For more on the background of these strategies, see David Osborne and Ted Gaebler, *Reinventing Government* (Reading, Mass.: Addison-Wesley, 1992). See also Hindy Lauer Schachter, *Reinventing Government or Reinventing Ourselves* (Albany: State University of New York Press, 1996).

16. It is important to note that Congress had specifically separated implementation of the ADA for outdoor developed areas from implementation for federal wilderness areas. The National Council on Disability was given the task of conducting a study and report on the effect that wilderness designation and land management practices have on the ability of individuals with disabilities to enjoy wilderness areas. See *Congressional Record—Senate*, September 7, 1989, 19833.

17. Unapproved meeting minutes, Outdoor Regulatory Negotiation Committee on Outdoor Developed Areas, Washington, D.C., June 26–27, 1997.

18. Cynthia D. Waddell, "Applying the ADA to the Internet: A Web Accessibility Standard," available at www.icdri.org (January 30, 2001).

19. Ibid.

20. "Board Issues Standards for Electronic and Information Technology," *Access Currents* 6, no. 6 (November–December 2000): 1.

21. "Update on Standards for Electronic and Information Technology," *Access Currents*, 6 no. 5 (September–October 2000): 2.

22. Exemplary of the discussion is an article by Susan Webb, "The Debate over ADAAG," *Mainstream* (November 1997): 30–35.

23. "Board Marks ADA's 10th Anniversary with Public Forum," *Access Currents* 6, no. 4 (July–August 2000): 1.

24. "Board Works to Advance Standards on Classroom Acoustics," *Access Currents* 7, no. 6 (November–December 2001): 1.

25. "The Access Board: Enforcing Accessible Design for 25 Years (1976–2001)," *Access Currents* 7, no. 3 (May–June 2001): 3.

26. Frank D. Roylance, "Warship to Offer Access to Decks," *Baltimore Sun* (February 2, 1999), B1.

27. Van Meter and Van Horn, "The Policy Implementation Process," 467–68.

28. National Council on Disability, *Achieving Independence: The Challenge for the 21st Century: A Decade of Progress in Disability Policy, Setting an Agenda for the Future* (Washington, D.C.: National Council on Disability, 1996), 155.

29. National Council on Disability, *Enforcing the Civil Rights of Air Travelers with Disabilities* (Washington, D.C.: National Council on Disability, 1999).

30. National Council on Disability, *Back to School on Civil Rights* (Washington, D.C.: National Council on Disability, 1999).

31. National Council on Disability, *Promises to Keep: A Decade of Federal Enforcement of the Americans with Disabilities Act* (Washington, D.C.: National Council on Disability, 2000).

32. Ibid., 9.

33. Ibid., 13.

34. Ruth Colker, "ADA Title II: A Fragile Compromise," in Francis and Silvers, *Exploring Implications*, 302.

35. *Settlement Agreement Between the United States of America and the Oakland Police Department*, April 7, 1998.

36. *Howe v. Hull*, No. 3:92CV7658 (Ohio, 1994).

37. See, for example, *Perry v. Command Performance*, 913 F.2d 99 (3rd Cir. 1990), in which a black woman was refused service by a beauty salon, or *Perry v. Burger King Corp.*, 924 F. Supp. 548 (1996), in which a restaurant refused to allow the plaintiff to use a restroom.

38. "Two Hotel Chains Agree on Guaranteed Rooms for Disabled," *San Francisco Chronicle* (December 17, 1998), A16.

39. "National Settlement Agreement Reached in Americans with Disabilities Act Lawsuit," press release, Disability Rights Education and Defense Fund, June 18, 1998.

40. Colker, "ADA Title II," 305.

41. Mary Johnson, "Montana Resort Fights Access," *Ragged Edge* (March 3, 2002), available at www.raggededgemagazine.com/extra/barredas.

42. See Arlene B. Mayerson, "What Is DREDF?" *ADA Gala*, February 1, 1992, 6–9.

43. Laurence W. Paradis, "Disability Rights Laws: No Better than Their Enforcement," *New Mobility* (January 1998), available at www.newmobility.com/review_article.cfm?id=73&action=browse

44. Marc Galanter, "Why the Haves Come Out Ahead: Speculations on the Limits of Social Change," *Law and Society Review* 9 (1974): 95–160.

45. Donald R. Songer and Reginald S. Sheehan, "Who Wins on Appeal? Upperdogs and Underdogs in the United States Courts of Appeals," *American Journal of Political Science* 36 (1992): 235–58.

46. Donald R. Songer, Ashlyn Kuersten, and Erin Kaheny, "Why the Haves Don't Always Come Out Ahead: Repeat Players Meet *Amici Curiae* for the Disadvantaged," *Political Research Quarterly* 53, no. 3 (September 2000): 537–56.

47. Paradis, "Disability Rights Laws."

48. Thayer C. Scott, "Disabled Woman, Alameda Depot Settle Bias Suit," *San Francisco Chronicle* (November 27, 1997), A25.

49. *Kimel v. Florida Board of Regents*, 120 S.Ct. 631 (2000).

50. *Crowder v. Kitagawa*, 81 F.3d. 1480 (9th Cir. 1996).

51. Richard Scotch, *From Good Will to Civil Rights: Transforming Federal Disability Policy* (Philadelphia: Temple University Press, 1984), 1.

52. See, for example, Richard A. Epstein, *Forbidden Grounds: The Case against Employment Discrimination Laws* (Cambridge, Mass.: Harvard University Press, 1992), and compare with Michael Ashley Stein, "Market Failure and ADA Title I," in Francis and Silvers, *Americans with Disabilities,* 193–98, or Peter David Blanck, *The Americans with Disabilities Act and the Emerging Workforce* (Washington, D.C.: American Association on Mental Retardation, 1998).

53. Peter David Blanck, "Studying Disability, Employment Policy and the ADA," in Francis and Silvers, *Americans with Disabilities,* 212.

54. U.S.C. 12102(2); 29 C.F.R. 1630.2(g).

55. *Carlson v. Inacom Corp.*, 885 Supp. 1314 (D. Nebraska 1995).

56. *Siefken v. Village of Arlington Heights*, 65 F.3d 664 (7th Cir. 1995).

57. S. Ct. 2133 (1999).

58. Arlene Mayerson and Matthew Diller, "The Supreme Court's Near-Sighted View of the ADA," e-mail correspondence to berkeley-disabled@netcom.com, 13 July 1999.

59. Ibid.

60. *Matthews v. Jefferson*, 29 F. Supp 2d 525 (W.D. Ark. 1998).

61. *Soto v. City of Newark*, 72 F. Supp 2d 489 (D.N.J. 1999).

62. *McGregor v. National Railroad Passenger Corp.*, 187 F.3d 1113 (9th Cir. 1999).

63. Ibid., 9–10.

64. Patricia Illingworth and Wendy E. Parmet, "Positively Disabled: The Relationship between the Definition of Disability and Rights under the ADA," in Francis and Silvers, *Americans with Disabilities,* 9.

65. Ibid., 11.

66. Personal correspondence to author, April 11, 2001.

Chapter 7

1. See, for example, Florence P. Haseltine, Sandra S. Cole, and David B. Gray, eds., *Reproductive Issues for Persons with Physical Disabilities* (Baltimore: Paul H. Brookes, 1993); Lynette Lamb, "Selecting for Perfection: Is Prenatal Screening Becoming a Kind of Eugenics?" *Utne Reader* 66 (November–December 1994), 26–28.

2. Adrienne S. Asch, "The Human Genome and Disability Rights," *Disability Rag and Resource* (January–February 1994), 12–15.

3. A group of disability studies scholars also submitted a rebuttal to the Hastings Report. *The Disability Rights Critique of Prenatal Genetic Testing: Reflections and Recommendations* (Garrison, N.Y.: The Hastings Center, 1999).

4. "Wrongful Life," *Ragged Edge* 1 (2001), 49.

5. *Procanik v. Cillo*, 478 A.2d 755 (N.J. 1984).

6. Lori B. Andrews and Michelle Hibbert, "Courts and Wrongful Birth: Can Disability Itself Be Viewed as a Legal Wrong?" in *Americans with Disabilities: Exploring Implications of the Law for Individuals and Institutions,* ed. Leslie Pickering Francis and Anita Silvers (New York: Routledge, 2000), 318.

7. See Erik Parens and Adrienne Asch, eds., *Prenatal Testing and Disability Rights* (Washington, D.C.: Georgetown University Press, 2000).

8. Lisa Blumberg, "The Bad Baby Blues: Reproductive Technology and the Threat to Diversity," *Ragged Edge* (July–August 1998): 16.

9. "Conflicted," *Ragged Edge* 1 (2001): 46.

10. Abby Lippman, "The Genetic Construction and Prenatal Testing: Choice, Consent, or Conformity for Women?" in *Women and Prenatal Testing: Facing the Challenges of Genetic Technology,* ed. Karen H. Rothenberg and Elizabeth Thomson (Athens: Ohio University Press, 1994), 15.

11. Andrews and Hibbert, "Courts and Wrongful Birth," 327, 321.

12. See, for example, *Becker v. Schwartz*, 386 N.E.2d 807 (1978); *Haymon v. Wilkerson,* 555 Acted 880 (D.C. 1987); and *Naccash v. Burg*, 290 S.E.2d 825 (Va. 1982).

13. The case of Oregon is almost always used to illustrate this point. See, for example, David Orentlicher, "Rationing and the Americans with Disabilities Act," *Journal of the American Medical Association* 271 (1994): 308–14, and Dan W. Brock, "Health Care Resource Prioritization and Discrimination against Persons with Disabilities," in Francis and Silvers, *Americans with Disabilities*, 223–35.

14. Margaret P. Battin, Rosamond Rhodes, and Anita Silvers, eds., *Physician Assisted Suicide: Expanding the Debate* (New York: Routledge, 1998).

15. Elaine Fox, Jeffrey J. Kamakahi, and Stella M. Capek, *Come Lovely and Soothing Death: The Right to Die Movement in the United States* (New York: Twayne Publishers, 1999), 26.

16. Elisabeth Kubler-Ross, *On Death and Dying* (New York: Macmillian, 1969).

17. Barney Glaser and Anselm Strauss, *Awareness of Dying* (Chicago: Aldine, 1975).

18. Paul K. Longmore, "Elizabeth Bouvia, Assisted Suicide and Social Prejudice," *Issues in Law and Medicine* 3, no. 2 (fall 1987): 141–68.

19. *Washington v. Glucksberg,* 117 S.Ct. 2258 (1997); *Vacco v. Quill,* 117 S.Ct. 2293 (1997).

20. Fox, Kamakahi and Capek, *Come Lovely and Soothing Death,* 27–28.

21. Derek Humphry, *Let Me Die before I Wake* (Eugene, Ore.: Hemlock Society, 1981).

22. Derek Humphrey, *Final Exit* (New York: Harper and Row, 1991).

23. For examples of disability activists' views, see the January/February/March 1997 issue of *Mouth: The Voice of Disability Rights*, particularly its coverage of demonstrations before the U.S. Supreme Court.

24. Ricky Young, "Ten Euthanasia Foes Charged," *Denver Post Online* (January 24, 1998); available at www.denverpost.online.

25. Oregon Death with Dignity Act, ORS Section 127.800-127-897.

26. A. E. Chin and others, "Legalized Physician-Assisted Suicide in Oregon—The First Year's Experience," *New England Journal of Medicine* 340 (1999): 577–83.

27. "People Killed Selves in 2000 under Oregon Law," *Arizona Republic* (February 22, 2001), A-6.

28. Lois Snyder and Arthur Caplan, "Assisted Suicide: Finding Common Ground," *Annals of Internal Medicine* 132, no. 6 (March 21, 2000): 468–69.

29. "Death with Dignity Dies a Quiet Death in California," *Ragged Edge* (March–April 2000), 8.

30. "British Medical Journal Lauds Kevorkian as 'Hero,'" *Detroit News* (June 9, 1996); available at www.detnews.com (accessed November 19, 2001).

31. "Not Dead Yet Angered at Kevorkian Award," *Ragged Edge* (May–June 2000), 9.

32. "Peter Singer Appointment Draws Warning," *Ragged Edge* (September–October 1998), 9.

33. Katha Pollit, "Peter Singer Comes to Princeton," *The Nation* 268, no. 16 (May 3, 1999): 10.

34. "Disability Scholar Says Singer Views 'Misguided,'" *Ragged Edge* (November–December 1999), 3–4.

35. Evan Kemp, Jr., "Aiding the Disabled: No Pity, Please," *New York Times* (September 3, 1981).

36. Leslie Bennetts, "Jerry vs. the Kids," www.eka.com/evan/jerry/ (November 26, 2000).

37. "Telethon's (Embarrassing) Moments," www.tvparty.com/embarrass (January 31, 2001). The comment is part of a "classic moments in television" video advertisement.

38. Jerry Lewis, "If I Had Muscular Dystrophy," *Parade* (September 2, 1990).

39. Bennetts, "Jerry vs. the Kids."

40. "Ragged Edge Extra," www.raggededgemagazine.com/extra/jerrylewis (March 5, 2002).

41. Bennetts, "Jerry vs. the Kids."

42. Steven E. Brown, "Super Duper: The (Unfortunate) Ascendancy of Christopher Reeve and the Cure-All for the 1990s," *Mainstream* 21, no. 2 (October 1996): 28–31. See also Sam Maddox, "Christopher Reeve: Making Sense Out of Chaos," *New Mobility* 7, no. 35 (August 1996): 58–66, 104–5.

43. Pat Williams, "Christopher Reeve: What's It Gonna Take?" *The Electric Edge* (January–February 1997), 17; available at www.ragged-edge-mag.com/archive/plbstory.

44. Ibid.

45. "Christopher Reeve Named Vice Chairman of the National Organization on Disability," press release, National Organization on Disability (June 3, 1997); available at www.nod.org/press.

46. Michelle Malkin, "Battles against Disease Are Overpoliticized," www.townhall.com/columnists (March 12, 2000). See also Wolf Blitzer, "The Impact of Celebrity Fund Raising," *Capitol Times* 2, no. 44 (September 30, 1999); available at www.capitoltimes.com.

47. Ibid.

48. Joseph P. Shapiro, *No Pity: People with Disabilities Forging a New Civil Rights Movement* (New York: Random House, 1993), 99.

49. See, for example, Arden Neisser, *The Other Side of Silence: Sign Language and the Deaf Community in America* (New York: Knopf, 1983).

50. Charlotte Baker and Carol Paden, *American Sign Language: A Look at Its History, Structure, and Community* (Silver Spring, Md.: T. J. Publishers, 1978).

51. See Harry Best, *Deafness and the Deaf in the United States* (New York: Macmillan, 1943).

52. This perspective comes from Karen Nakamura, whose website offers insights on Deaf culture to those she calls "deaf-impaired." See www.deaflibrary.org.

53. For more on the portrayal of deafness, see Martin F. Norden, *The Cinema of Isolation: A History of Physical Disability in the Movies* (New Brunswick, N.J.: Rutgers University Press, 1994), and Matthew Scott Moore and Robert F. Panara, *Great Deaf Americans* (Rochester, N.Y.: Deaf Life Press, 1996).

54. See Jerome D. Schein, *At Home among Strangers* (Washington, D.C.: Gallaudet University Press, 1989), and Harlan Lane, *When the Mind Hears: A History of the Deaf* (New York: Random House, 1984).

55. See, for example, Marian Corker, "The U.K. Disability Discrimination Act," in Francis and Silvers, *Americans with Disabilities*, 357–62.

56. Carol Padden and Tom Humphries, *Deaf in America: Voices from a Culture* (Cambridge, Mass.: Harvard University Press, 1988).

57. Shapiro, *No Pity*, 100–104.

58. See, for example, "Deaf Man's Hearing Restored by Implant," *Silent News* (September 1996), 28.

59. "Cochlear Implants in Adults and Children," NIH Consensus Statement Online, May 15–17, 1995 cited February 2, 2001; vol. 13, no. 2, 1–30.

60. The militancy and inflammatory rhetoric of those opposed to the cochlear implant, especially for children, is widespread.

61. Samantha Yaffe, "To Hear or Not to Hear," *Toronto Sun* (March 7, 1999), available at www.deafworldweb.org/pub.

62. "Cochlear Implants: The Final Putdown?" *Disability Rag and Resource* (March–April 1986), 1, 4–6.

63. Owen Wrigley, *The Politics of Deafness* (Washington, D.C.: Gallaudet University Press, 1996), 211–12.

64. NAD position statement on cochlear implants, July 16, 2001; available at www.nad.org/infocenter/newsroom/positions.

65. Ibid.

66. Nancy J. Bloch, "Cochlear Implants and the NAD," *NAD Broadcaster* (January 2001), available at www.nad.org/infocenter/infotogo/dcc (accessed July 16, 2001).

67. Linda Greenhouse, "Pivotal Rulings Ahead: Supreme Court to Begin Review of Americans with Disabilities Act," *New York Times* (April 19, 1999).

68. "*Olmstead* Attacks the ADA via the Supremes," e-mail correspondence sent December 23, 1998.

69. Ibid.

70. Mary Johnson, "Bed Money," *Ragged Edge* (May–June 2000), 10–15, 25, 29.

71. Wendy Fox-Grage and others, *The States' Response to the* Olmstead *Decision: A Work in Progress* (Washington, D.C.: National Conference of State Legislatures, 2002).

72. Lois and Elaine, "Free at Last," *Ragged Edge* (September–October 2000), 8.

73. Bernard Lefkowitz, *Our Guys: The Glen Ridge Rape and the Secret Life of the Perfect Suburb* (Berkeley: University of California Press, 1997).

74. Leora Tanenbaum, "Boys Town," *Salon* (August 13, 1997).

75. See also Peter Laufer, *A Question of Consent: Innocence and Complicity in the Glen Ridge Rape Case* (San Francisco: Mercury House, 1994), and Richard Sobsey, *Violence and Abuse in the Lives of People with Disabilities: The End of Silent Acceptance?* (Baltimore: Paul H. Brookes, 1994).

76. Hate crimes legislation, n.d., available at www.nvc.org/ddir (accessed June 30, 1998).

77. Ibid.

78. U.S.C. 994, Section 280003(a) of the Violent Crime Control and Law Enforcement Act of 1994.

79. Daniel D. Sorenson, *The Invisible Victims* (Minneapolis: Institute on Community Integration, 1996).

80. Dick Sobsey and T. Doe, "Patterns of Sexual Abuse and Disability," *Sexuality and Disability* 9 (1991): 243–59.

81. Barbara Faye Waxman, "Hatred: The Unacknowledged Dimension in Violence against Disabled People," *Journal of Sexuality and Disability* 9, no. 3 (October–November 1991): 261–71; idem, "Hate," *Disability Rag and Resource* 13, no. 3 (May–June 1992): 4–7; Sobsey, *Violence and Disability.*

82. Barbara Faye Waxman and Leslie R. Wolfe, *Violence against Disabled Women* (Washington, D.C.: Center for Women Policy Studies, 1999).

83. Kimberle Crenshaw, "Demarginalizing The Intersection of Race and Sex: A Black Feminist Critique of Anti-Discrimination Doctrine, Feminist Theory, and Antiracist Politics," in *Living with Contradiction: Controversies in Feminist Social Ethics,* ed. Allison Jaggar (Boulder, Colo.: Westview, 1994), 40.

84. Lennard J. Davis, "Go to the Margins of the Class," in Francis and Silvers, *Americans with Disabilities,* 333.

85. Waxman and Wolfe, *Violence against Disabled Women.*

86. Equal Employment Opportunity Commission, *EEOC Enforcement Guidance on the Americans with Disabilities Act and Psychiatric Disabilities,* www.eeoc.gov/docs (accessed March 1, 2001).

87. Ibid.

88. Ibid.

89. Ibid.

90. *Miller v. National Cas. Co.,* 61 F.3d 627 (8th Cir. 1995).

91. Rhonda Zwillinger, "No Safe Haven," *E Magazine* 9, no. 5 (September–October 1998); available at www.emagazine.com (accessed June 12, 2001). See also "Multiple Chemical Sensitivity," Arizona Technology Access Program (n.d.), and Lynn Lawson, *Staying Well in a Toxic World: Understanding Environmental Illness, Multiple Chemical Sensitivity, Chemical Injuries, and Sick Building Syndrome* (Evanston, Ill.: Lynn Lawson, 1993).

92. "Ecology House: Evaluation and List of Building Materials," www.users.lanminds.com (accessed June 12, 2001).

93. "Deceptive Draft Report on Multiple Chemical Sensitivity Released for Public Comment by U.S. Federal Interagency Workshop on MCS," press release, MCS Referral and Resources (September 9, 1998).

94. "Excessive Use of Fragrance Products in Public Places," San Francisco Bay chapter, Sierra Club, Conservation Committee, Resolution 98.12.01, December 1998.

CHAPTER 8

1. National Organization on Disability, *The State of the Union 2002 for Americans with Disabilities* (Washington, D.C.: National Organization on Disability, 2002); available at www.nod.org (accessed July 5, 2002).

2. Most of the evaluations were conducted during the first few years after the ADA's passage. See, for example, Peter C. Bishop and Augustus J. Jones, Jr., "Implementing the Americans with Disabilities Act of 1990: Assessing the Variables of Success," *Public Administration Review* 53, no. 2 (March-April 1993): 121–28; Frederick C. Collignon, "Is the ADA Successful? Indicators for Tracking Gains," *Annals of the American Academy of Political and Social Science* 549 (January 1997): 129–47.

3. Executive summary, *Survey Program on Participation and Attitudes* (Washington, D.C.: National Organization on Disability, 2001); available at www.nod.org/hs2000 (accessed July 5, 2001).

4. "New Harris Survey Marks Strong Approval for ADA Nine Years after Passage," press release, National Organization on Disability (April 15, 1999); available at www.nod.org/press.

5. Ibid.

6. Ibid.

7. Center for Research on Women with Disabilities press release (July 7, 1997), available at www.bcm.tmc.edu/crowd (accessed November 19, 1997); Ellen W. Grabois and Margaret A. Nosek, "The Americans with Disabilities Act and Medical Providers: Ten Years after Passage of the Act," *Policy Studies Journal*, 29, no. 4 (2001): 682–89.

8. Personal correspondence to author, January 16, 1999.

9. Executive summary, *Survey Program on Participation and Attitudes*.

10. Ibid.

11. John M. McNei,. "Employment, Earnings, and Disability," paper prepared for Seventy-Fifth Annual Conference of Western Economic Association International, Vancouver, British Columbia, June 29–July 3, 2000.

12. U.S. Census Bureau, *Statistical Abstract of the United States: 2000* (Washington, D.C.: U.S. Government Printing Office, 2000), 415.

13. "President Clinton and Vice President Gore Unveil New Initiative to Improve Economic Opportunities for Americans with Disabilities," press release (January 13, 1999).

14. U.S. Department of Labor press release (February 9 2000), available at www.dol.gov/opa (accessed November 2, 2000); Tony Coehlo, farewell letter, President's Committee on Employment of People with Disabilities (October 9, 2000), available at www.pcepd.gov (accessed November 2, 2000).

15. "EEOC Files Third Disability-Based Discrimination Suit against Northwest," Disability News Service, www.disabilitynews.com (accessed June 12, 2001).

16. National Organization on Disability, *State of the Union 2002*.

17. Kay Schriner and Andrew Batavia," The Americans with Disabilities Act: Does It Secure the Fundamental Right to Vote?" *Policy Studies Journal* 29, no. 4 (2001): 663–73.

18. Kay Schriner, Lisa A. Ochs, and Todd G. Shields, "The Last Suffrage Movement: Voting Rights for Persons with Cognitive and Emotional Disabilities," *Publius* 27, no. 3 (summer 1997): 75–96.

19. Steve Bousquet, "Disabled Seek Greater Voice in New Voting Method," *St. Petersburg Times Online* (July 25, 2001); available at www.sptimes.com/News/072501.

20. "Disabled Philadelphians Sue City for Right to Vote," press release, National Organization on Disability; available at www,nod.org (accessed June 12, 2001). See also "Voters with Disabilities Face Discrimination Nationwide," *Ragged Edge* (November–December 2000), 5–7.

21. "The Disability Vote in the November 2000 Presidential Election," National Organization on Disability (August 3, 2001), available at www.nod.org/cont (accessed July 5, 2002).

22. "Election Reform: Include Voter Access!" www.jfanow.org, n.d. (accessed April 11, 2001).

23. U.S. General Accounting Office (GAO), *Voters with Disabilities: Access to Polling Places and Alternative Voting Methods* (Washington, D.C.: U.S. General Accounting Office, 2001).

24. For the history and implementation of the statute, see Frances Fox Piven and Richard A. Cloward, *Why Americans Still Don't Vote* (Boston: Beacon Press, 2000).

25. Ibid., 265.

26. U.S. GAO, *Voters with Disabilities*, 7.

27. Personal correspondence to author, April 21, 1999.

28. Personal correspondence to author, November 2, 1999.

29. Personal correspondence to author, May 24, 1999.

30. See Ronald L. Mace, Graeme J. Hardie, and Jaine P. Place, "Accessible Environments: Toward Universal Design," in *Design Intervention: Toward a More Humane Architecture,* ed. Wolfgang F. E. Preiser and others (New York: Van Nostrand Reinhold, 1991); and Wolfgang F. E. Prieser and Elaine Ostroff, eds., *Universal Design Handbook* (New York: McGraw-Hill, 1991)

31. Ronald L. Mace, Graeme J. Hardie, and Jaine P. Place, "Excerpts from Accessible Environments," www.design.ncsu.edu/cud/pubs, n.d. (accessed July 23, 2001).

32. Jim Davis, "Design for the 21st Century Starts Now," *Ragged Edge* (November–December 1998), 10–14.

33. Fred Pelka, *The Disability Rights Movement* (Santa Barbara, Calif.: ABC-CLIO, 1997), 30.

34. "Closed Captions and Descriptive Narration Available for First Time as Part of Feature Film Presentation," press release, National Center for Accessible Media (November 21, 1997).

35. "Wells Fargo, California Council of the Blind Announce Nation's First Plan for Talking ATMs," joint press release (June 23, 1999).

36. John Williams, "Section 508: A Mandate for Technological Accessibility," National Organization on Disability, n.d.; available at www.nod.org/williams (accessed June 12, 2001).

37. Cynthia D. Waddell, "Understanding the Digital Economy," available at www.icdri.org (accessed June 7, 2000).

38. Ibid.

39. American Library Association, *The 1998 National Survey of U.S. Public Library Outlet Internet Connectivity: Final Report* (Washington, D.C.: American Library Association, 1998).

40. Stephanie Thomas, Foreward, in *To Ride the Public's Buses: The Fight that Built a Movement,* ed. Mary Johnson and Barrett Shaw (Louisville, Ky.: Advocado Press, 2001), viii.

41. Timothy M. Cook, "The Americans with Disabilities Act: The Move to Integration," *Temple Law Review* 64 (1991): 420.

42. *Henderson v. United States,* 339 U.S. 816 (1950).

43. Cook, "The Americans with Disabilities Act: The Move to Integration," 424.

44. Executive summary, *Survey Program on Participation and Attitudes.*

45. National Organization on Disability, *State of the Union 2002.*

46. "DOT commits to accessibility with new policies and programs," personal correspondence to author (September 29, 1999).

47. "Greyhound to Improve Bus Service to Passengers under Justice Department Agreement," press release, U.S. Department of Justice (September 30, 1999); available at www.usdog.opa/pr (accessed July 29, 2001).

48. National Organization on Disability, *State of the Union 2002.*

49. U.S. Surgeon General, *Closing the Gap: A National Blueprint to Improve the Health of Persons with Mental Retardation* (February 2002), available at (www.surgeongeneral.gov/topics/mentalretardation (accessed July 6, 2002).

50. "America's People with Disabilities Need the MiCASSA in 1999," www.tash.org/govaffairs/support_micassa_now (accessed July 14, 2001).

51. Larry Biondi, "A 'Lifeline' Makes Slow Progress in Congress," *Ragged Edge* 3 (2001): 7.

52. Mary Johnson, "In Thrall to the Medical Model," *Ragged Edge* (January–February 1999), 14.

53. "Sea Change: Finally the Money Is Starting to 'Follow the Person,'" *Ragged Edge* 4 (2001): 8.

54. Mary Johnson, "Bed Money," *Ragged Edge* (May–June 2000), 13.

55. Lawrence O. Gostin, "Impact of the ADA on the Health Care System," in *Implementing the Americans with Disabilities Act,* ed. Lawrence O. Gostin and Henry A. Beyer (Baltimore: Paul H. Brookes, 1993), 180.

56. Barbara A. Crowley, "Rolling in the Emergency Room," *Ragged Edge* (July–August 2000), 17–18, 20; Rus Cooper-Dowda, "Alice in Emergencyroom Land," *Ragged Edge Online,* www.raggededgemagazine.com/extra/aliceERland (accessed July 6, 2002).

57. H. Stephen Kaye, *Disability Watch: The Status of People with Disabilities in the United States* (Volcano, Calif.: Volcano Press, 1997), 56.

58. "Access to Single-Family Homes Moves Closer in Illinois, Arizona," *Ragged Edge* 2/3 (2002): 7.

59. National Council on Disability, *Promises to Keep: A Decade of Federal Enforcement of the Americans with Disabilities Act* (Washington, D.C.: National Council on Disability, 2000).

60. Ibid.

61. Ibid.

62. Stephen L. Percy, "Challenges and Dilemmas in Implementing the Americans with Disabilities Act: Lessons from the First Decade," *Policy Studies Journal* 29, no. 4 (2001): 633–40.

63. Collignon, "Is the ADA Successful?" 139.

64. 2000 NOD/Harris survey of Americans with disabilities, executive summary; available at www.nod.org/hs2000 (accessed July 5, 2001).

65. Anthony Downs, "Up and Down with Ecology—The 'Issue-Attention Cycle,'" *The Public Interest* 28 (summer 1972): 38–50.

EPILOGUE

1. Anne Gearan, "Disabilities Law Flawed, O'Connor Says," *Arizona Republic* (March 15, 2002).

2. Nos. CV-97-AR-92-S and CV-97-AR-2179-S; 989 F. Supp. 1409 (N.D. Ala. 1998).

3. Ibid.

4. 193 F 3d 1214 (1999).

5. The states are Arizona, Connecticut, Illinois, Iowa, Kentucky, Maryland, Massachusetts, Minnesota, Missouri, New Mexico, New York, North Dakota, Vermont, and Washington.

6. G. Wayne Barr, "Case Imperils Protection of Disability Rights," *National Catholic Reporter* 36 (October 6, 2000): 22.

7. "Brief of Morton Horwitz, Martha Field, Martha Minow, and over 100 Other Historians and Scholars, *Amici Curiae* in Support of Respondents"; available at www.raggededgemagazine.com/garrett (accessed October 5, 2000).

8. Ala. Code tit.45, ch. 6, Section 239.

9. 1904 Md. Laws, art. 59, Section 1.

10. 89 ILL. COMP. STAT. Section 2 (1916).

11. 1913 Mich. Public Acts, No. 34; 1925 Minn. Laws 140, ch. 154.

12. Miss. Code. Ann. Section 41-21-45 (1990).

13. "Brief of Lambda Legal Defense and Education Fund, Inc. et al., *Amici Curiae* in Support of Respondents," available at www.aclu.org/court/garrett (accessed February 8, 2001).

14. "The *Garrett* Case: New Challenge to the ADA," Bazelon Center for Mental Health Law (October 8, 2000); available at www.bazelon.org/garrettcase (accessed February 11, 2001).

15. "Statement of Former President George H. W. Bush as *Amicus Curiae* in Support of Respondents," available at www.bazelon.org/presidentbushbrief (accessed March 1, 2001).

16. "Statement by National Council on Disability Chairperson Marca Bristo on the U.S. Supreme Court Case, *University of Alabama v. Garrett*," NCD#01-314, October 3, 2000; available at www.ncd.gov/newsroom/news/r01-314 (accessed February 11, 2001).

17. A transcript is available at www.supremecourtus.gov/calendar/argument_trans.

18. *Kimel v. Florida Bd. of Regents*, 120 S. Ct. 631 (2000).

19. This comment, and the others that follow, are interpreted from *Board of Trustees of the University of Alabama, et al., v. Patricia Garrett, et al.*, 531 U.S. 356 (2001).

20. The rational-basis scrutiny had been established in *Cleburne v. Cleburne Living Center, Inc.*, 473 U.S. 432 (1985). That case involved an equal protection challenge to a city ordinance requiring a special use permit for the operation of a group home for mentally retarded people.

21. This view previously had been noted in *City of Boerne v. Flores*, 521 U.S. 507 (1997).

22. Somewhat ironically, two attorneys writing two months before the decision was handed down said there was little likelihood that the state of Alabama would prevail in the case, writing, "The ADA is not dead." See John W. Griffin Jr., and Bob D. Brown, "Chipping Away at the ADA," *Trial* 36 (December 2000): 48.

23. "States above the Law," *Washington Post* (February 24, 2001), A22.

24. E. J. Dionne, Jr., "The Overreaching Court," *Washington Post* (February 23, 2001), A23.

25. Linda Greenhouse, "Justices Give the States Immunity from Suits by Disabled Workers," *New York Times* (February 23, 2001).

26. "National Council on Disability Deeply Troubled by U.S. Supreme Court Decision Limiting Scope of Americans with Disabilities Act," press

release, National Council on Disability (February 21, 2001); available at www.ncd.gov/newsroom/news/ (accessed February 27, 2001).

27. "Disability Rights Advocates Respond to Supreme Court *Garrett* Ruling," www.raggededgemagazine.com/drn/garrettadawatchresp (accessed February 27, 2001).

28. "In Disappointing Decision, Justices Limit Disability Law," press release, American Civil Liberties Union (February 21, 2001); available at www.aclu.org/news/2001 (accessed March 1, 2001).

29. "American Association of People with Disabilities Blasts Supreme Court Ruling Limiting ADA," www.aapd-dc.org/docs/garrett (accessed February 27, 2001).

30. "Disability Rights Advocates Respond," www.raggededgemagazine.com/drn/garrettadawatchresp.

31. "The Arc of the United States 'Disappointed' in Divided Court's Decision Limiting the Scope of the ADA," www.thearc.org/garrett (accessed February 27, 2001).

32. "Supreme Court Rules 5–4 to Limit ADA in Garrett Decision," www.raggededgemagazine.com/drn/drn (accessed February 27, 2001).

33. See "Remarks by the President in Announcement of New Freedom Initiative," White House press release (February 1, 2001); available at www.whitehouse.gov/news/releases (accessed March 1, 2001); "New Freedom Initiative for People with Disabilities," www.disabilityworld.org (accessed February 28, 2001).

34. "Investing in Independence: Transition Recommendations for President George W. Bush," National Council on Disability, January 2001; available at www.ncd.gov/newsroom/publications/bush (accessed March 1, 2001).

35. The three cases on appeal were *Brown v. North Carolina*, 99-424, *California v. Dare*, 99-1417, and *Neinast v. Texas*, 00-263.

36. "Justices Sidestep Disabled Parking Tags Dispute," www.cnn.com/2001/LAW (accessed February 28, 2001).

37. *United States v. Snyder*, 00-554.

38. "Justices Decline to Take on Disabilities Law," www.cnn.com/2001/LAW (accessed February 28, 2001).

39. *Martin v. PGA Tour, Inc.*, 984 F.Supp.1242 (Ore. 1998).

40. 204 F. 3d 994 (2000).

41. *PGA Tour, Inc. v. Casey Martin*, 532 U.S. 661 (2001), at 29.

42. "Casey Courageous," *Ragged Edge* 4 (2001), 4, 50.

43. "NOD Reaction to the Supreme Court's Casey Martin Decision," www.nod.org (accessed July 5, 2001).

44. "CNN's Charles Bierbauer on the Martin Ruling," www.sportsillustrated.cnn.com (accessed July 5, 2001).

45. Dave Kindred, "One Man, Standing Tall," *Sporting News* (February 9, 1998), 2.

46. Dissent of Justice Scalia, *PGA Tour, Inc. v. Casey Martin*, 532 U.S. 661 (2001).

47. "Dubya's New Podium—and New Policies," *Ragged Edge* 2 (2001): 4.

48. Radio address of the president to the nation, July 28, 2001; available at www.whitehouse.gov/news/releases (accessed July 29, 2001).

49. *Toyota Motor Mfg. v. Williams*, 122 S. Ct. 681 (2002).

50. James Vicini, "Supreme Court Narrows Reach of Disability Law," www.dailynews.yahoo.com (accessed January 8, 2002).

51. Christine Vargas, "Select Recent Court Decisions: Disability Law," *American Journal of Law and Medicine* 28 (2002): 124.

52. Ruth O'Brien, "The Supreme Court's Catch-22," www.raggededgemagazine.com/extra/obrienwilliams (accessed March 5, 2002).

53. Charles Lane, "Supreme Court Case Pits Disability against Seniority," *Washington Post* (December 5, 2001); available at www.washingtonpost.com/wp-dyn/articles (accessed February 13, 2002).

54. No. 00-1250 (2002).

55. "Supreme Court to Hear Arguments in ADA Employment Case *Echazabal v. Chevron*," www.accessiblesociety.org/topics/ada/echazabal1 (accessed March 5, 2002).

56. "Business Alert: Supreme Court Allows Employers to Deny Dangerous Jobs to Disabled Employees," U.S. Chamber of Commerce; available at www.uschamber.com/NCLC/Business1Alerts (accessed June 12, 2002).

57. "NCD Critical of Supreme Court Ruling," *Federal Human Resources Week* 9, no. 11 (2002); available at www.lexis-nexis.com/universe/document (accessed July 7, 2002).

58. No. 00-8452 (2002).

59. Ibid.

60. "AAMR Applauds U.S. Supreme Court Decision to Ban Execution of Persons with Mental Retardation," press release, American Association on Mental Retardation (June 20, 2002); available at www.aamr.org/Policies/death_penalty (accessed June 24, 2002).

61. Ruth O'Brien, *Crippled Justice: The History of Modern Disability Policy in the Workplace* (Chicago: University of Chicago Press, 2001), 220.

62. Ibid.

63. The coverage of the statue's unveiling and the Roosevelt quote are from Dave Reynolds, "Statue to Show 'Whole FDR,'" www.inclusiondaily.com/news/special/fdr (accessed March 5, 2002). See also Hugh Gregory Gallagher, *FDR in Photographs* (Clearwater, Fla.: Vandamere Press, 2001).

INDEX

Access Board, 59, 115, 118–25, 205
accessibility: ADA and, 118–25, 141; barriers to
independence and, 188–96; health care facilities and, 202–3; housing and, 203–5; outdoor,
120–22, 296n16; reg-neg process and, 120–22,
296n14; technology and, 122–24, 192–95; universal design, 174, 190–92; voting rights and,
181–82
Acoustical Society of America, 124–25
Act for the Relief of Sick and Disabled Seaman
(1798), 46
activism: ADA and, 6, 29, 77–79, 81–82, 84,
99–102, 184–85; civil rights model, 1, 9, 69–70,
74, 76, 83–84; coalition building, 77–79,
81–82, 84, 99–102, 184–85; cycles of issue
attention and, 207–8; debates over, 10–11, 13;
demonstrations and protests, 68–69, 80–86,
88, 153–54, 185; history of, 88–89; interest
groups and, 2, 6, 9, 71–74, 87–88, 133, 161–62,
185–87; litigation and, 29, 86–88, 133, 161–62;
militant, 6; post-ADA passage, 184–88,
228–30; as social movement, 3, 70–71, 74; as
"the splintered universe," 9, 76–77, 187–88
ADA Accessibility Guidelines (ADAAGs), 120,
121, 124
ADA Notification Act, 2, 278n2
ADAPT (American Disabled for Accessible
Public Transit), 80–82, 84, 108, 161–62, 173,
185, 189, 197, 200, 224
Advocacy, Inc., 87
advocacy groups. *See* interest groups
Age Discrimination in Employment Act, 137,
215
Aid to the Permanently and Totally Disabled
(1950), 51–52
Air Carriers Access Act (1986), 98–99, 197
Albertsons, Inc. v. Hallie Kirkinburg, 136, 140
Albrecht, Gary, 64–66
Alliance of Social Security Disability Recipients,
54–55

Alsbrook v. City of Maumelle, Arkansas, 135, 137
Altmeyer, Arthur, 49
American Association for Social Security, 48
American Association of People with
Disabilities, 91, 219
American Association on Mental Retardation
(AAMR), 228
American Civil Liberties Union, 101, 150, 213, 219
American Coalition of Citizens with
Disabilities, 84
American Council of the Blind, 77
American Hotel and Motel Association, 109–10
American Medical Association, 51, 101
American National Standards Institute (ANSI),
118, 124–25, 190
American Paralysis Association, 156
American Printing House for the Blind, 38
American Public Transit Association (APTA),
81, 110
American Red Cross, 66
American School for the Deaf (Hartford), 32, 157
American Sign Language (ASL), 39, 68, 156–57,
158
Americans with Disabilities Act (ADA) (1990):
accessibility and, 118–25, 141; amendments to,
2, 278n2; definition of disability, 5, 107,
139–40, 169, 178; employment and, 21, 113,
116–17, 128, 138, 141–42, 180, 192, 215;
enforcement, 126–28, 205–6; fusion of positive and negative rights, 142–43; implementation and rulemaking, 115–26, 160–64; integration mandate, 138–39, 160–64, 201–2; as
policy, 112–43; provisions of the law, 113–15;
Title I, 113, 116, 128, 138, 141–42, 180, 192, 215;
Title II, 113–14, 117, 129–30, 135, 181, 203–4,
215, 220–21; Title III, 114, 117, 118–25, 128,
130–31, 139–40, 204, 222; Title IV, 114; Title
V, 115. *See also* Americans with Disabilities
Act, litigation regarding; Americans with
Disabilities Act, passage of

311